SET ON EDGE

Your breakthrough step-by-step guide for conquering mental, women's, autoimmune, and metabolic health problems triggered by childhood distress, neglect, and trauma

DR. JANELLE LOUIS, ND

Set On Edge: Your breakthrough step-by-step guide for conquering mental, women's, autoimmune, and metabolic health problems triggered by childhood distress, neglect, and trauma

Copyright © 2019 Dr. Janelle Louis, ND. All rights reserved. No part of this book may be reproduced or transmitted in any form or by any means without written permission from the publisher.

Cover photo by Jeff Louis
Published by Focus Enterprises Publications, an imprint of Focus Integrative Healthcare LLC.

This book contains information relating to health and the care thereof. It is not intended to replace medical advice and should be used to supplement rather than replace regular care by your doctor. It is recommended that you seek your physician's advice before embarking on any medical program or treatment. All efforts have been made to ensure the accuracy of the information contained in this book as of the date of publication. The publisher and the author disclaim liability for any medical outcomes that may occur as a result of applying the methods described in this book. The statements in this book have not been evaluated by the FDA.

Publisher's Cataloging-in-Publication Data
Names: Louis, Janelle Aisha, author.
Title: Set on edge : your breakthrough step-by-step guide for conquering mental, women's, autoimmune, and metabolic health problems triggered by childhood distress, neglect, and trauma / Dr. Janelle Louis, ND.
Description: Includes bibliographical references. | Atlanta, GA: Focus Enterprises Publications, an imprint of Focus Integrative Healthcare LLC, 2019.
Identifiers: LCCN 2019917103 | ISBN 9780998350127
Subjects: LCSH Psychic trauma. | Psychic trauma in children--Complications. | Psychic trauma--Treatment. | Post-traumatic stress disorder. | Post-traumatic stress disorder in children--Complications. | Post-traumatic stress disorder--Treatment. | Adult child abuse victims--Health and hygiene. | Adult child abuse victims--Mental health. | Mind and body therapies. | BISAC SELF-HELP / Abuse | HEALTH & FITNESS / Alternative Therapies | PSYCHOLOGY / Psychopathology / Post-Traumatic Stress Disorder (PTSD)
Classification: LCC RC552.P67 .L68 2019 | DDC 616.8521--dc23

What's Your ACE Score?

Adverse Childhood Experiences, or childhood trauma, put you at risk. You may be up to 76% more likely to develop chronic disease as an adult depending on your ACE score. Approximately 1 in 2 people have experienced an ACE!

Make the life-chaning information I'll share profoundly meaningful and immediately useful by taking my free ACE quiz. It can't wait. Go to my site to get your ACE score now.

www.MyAceScore.com

CONTENTS

Preface 1

Introduction 5

CHAPTER 1: **Made For TV**
How ACEs found me before I was born and changed my life and family tree forever 9

CHAPTER 2: **Recently Found**
The sneaky culprit behind more than 30 diseases that you weren't paying attention to until now 21

CHAPTER 3: **Myth-buster**
The two most damaging myths that frustrate effective treatment, waste time and energy, and drain your emotions 41

CHAPTER 4: **Brain Strain**
How ACEs change your brain and create a breeding ground for mental health concerns in later life 55

CHAPTER 5: **Female Parts**
How ACEs increase risk for female health issues, reduce fertility, and keep you from enjoying the family you always pictured 71

CHAPTER 6:	**Friendly Fire**	
	How ACEs turn your immune system into a loose canon that's turned on itself	85
CHAPTER 7:	**Western Killers**	
	How fast food and sedentary lifestyles might not be the full story on the common killer diseases	101
CHAPTER 8:	**Find B.A.L.A.N.C.E.**	
	The ultimate guide to effective, comprehensive ACE treatment to help get on the road to recovery fast	117
CHAPTER 9:	**Dear Thriver**	
	Why ACEs don't have to define you, your future, or your dreams anymore	159

Appendix A: Explanation of My Dietary Recommendations 165

References 179

About the Author 193

To my two sons—for being my inspiration and my reasons for relentlessly pursuing my goal of eliminating the effects of childhood adversity on my life.

To my husband—for your compassion, your love, and your caring spirit. Thank you for being the love of my life and my partner on this ACE-defying journey. I love you eternally.

To my mother—for showing me that regardless of the traumatic events you've experienced, you can always bounce back and that, regardless of how ACEs have affected your life, it's never too late to make a positive change.

To my irreplaceable dad—for healing hearts you didn't break, loving children you didn't make, and teaching me by your example how a woman should be treated and what the term "fatherly love" truly means.

PREFACE

As I'll share in this book, adverse childhood experiences (ACEs) predispose us to four major categories of chronic disease. This includes mental health concerns like anxiety and depression, reproductive concerns like abnormal menstrual cycles and infertility, autoimmune diseases like lupus and rheumatoid arthritis, and metabolic concerns like diabetes, heart disease, and obesity. They also predispose us to some respiratory conditions and some forms of cancer. Yet very few physicians ask their patients about trauma history, and even fewer take childhood adversity into consideration when developing treatment plans.

For as long as I can remember, I've always been the type of person who asks *why*. When I learned about the link between childhood adversity and chronic disease, this didn't change. As a person who had experienced childhood adversity and who had seen its effects both on my own life and on the lives of my patients, I scoured the research to gain a clearer understanding of how exactly early life stress changes our physiology and affects our risk for chronic disease into adulthood. When I was finally able to make sense of the research to my satisfaction, I used that information to develop an integrative approach, the B.A.L.A.N.C.E. Framework™, which I then used to help my patients who had suffered childhood adversity to address their chronic health concerns and thrive. But something else happened… I found the experience of studying the research to be liberating. It was emotionally freeing to uncover physiological changes that had actually contributed to the person I had become. I was able to understand myself more and to extend more compassion to myself as a result.

As I continued to learn about the effects of ACEs, devouring study after study, I decided to share these resources with other survivors of childhood adversity so that they too could understand the scientific explanation for the symptoms they were experiencing and the diagnoses that they had been given. Unfortunately, however, I found the language in the research to be difficult to understand for non-medical professionals. I searched for other resources to share, but I couldn't find any that met my needs. I was searching for a resource that limited anecdotal evidence and gruesome details that could retraumatize those who read them. I wanted something that made the science easier to understand and that would provide its readers with hope and, most of all, with practical information on how to address the long-term effects of childhood adversity.

When I was unable to find such a resource, I decided to create my own. *Set On Edge* is the result. The title of this book was inspired by a Biblical proverb—the fathers have eaten sour grapes, and the children's teeth are *set on edge*. The proverb suggests that children are negatively impacted by their parents' choices and experiences. When this proverb is referenced in the Biblical text, however, it is quickly followed by the assertion that, from then on, there would be no more occasion for the use of this proverb. The children would no longer be negatively impacted by their parents' actions and experiences; the intergenerational nature of suffering would be no more. My desire to see this assertion accomplished is my motivation for writing this book.

I wrote this book in order to raise awareness about and limit the effects of childhood adversity, to help more people understand exactly how childhood adversity changes our brains and bodies, and to share the hopeful and promising message that despite our predispositions as survivors of childhood adversity, it isn't inevitable that we succumb to chronic disease in adulthood.

I wrote this book, *Set On Edge*, because it is my hope that, through education, more and more people will be able to break the cycle and eliminate the effects of ACEs on their own lives, that we'd have no more occasion to say, "She is this way because of what she experienced in childhood," but rather, "She is *this* way because of what she has overcome."

I wrote this book to share that it isn't too late, even for those of us who have already been diagnosed with ACE-related chronic conditions. With hard work, dedication, and my B.A.L.A.N.C.E. Framework™, which I'll be sharing, we can overcome the effects of early life stress and thrive.

It's my hope that this book effectively communicates this message to you.

INTRODUCTION

Before we get into the heart of the matter, there are a few things that I need you to understand. First of all, I need you to understand that I've written this book specifically for women because the people who seek my help in addressing their health concerns are overwhelmingly female and I'm most passionate about helping women. This doesn't mean that the principles found within this book will not be beneficial for male ACE survivors as well. In fact, with the exception of the female-specific information on reproductive concerns, I've used the principles I share in this book to help both female and male ACE survivors optimize their health and address ACE-related chronic diseases.

Second, if you are currently taking pharmaceutical medication to address your ACE-related chronic health concerns and you're content with your current solution, this book is not for you. This book was designed specifically for ACE-surviving women who aren't satisfied with their current health solutions and see a need for a different approach.

Maybe you're taking pharmaceutical medication to address your ACE-related chronic health concerns and you are unhappy with the side effects you're experiencing. Or maybe you're reluctant to start the medication you've been prescribed because you want to avoid medication-related side effects as much as possible. Perhaps you're taking medication, but your health is still out of control and you're just tired of your doctor increasing your dosage, adding on other medications, or changing your medication without seeing sufficient results. If one or more of these scenarios describes you and you feel like there must be a better way, *Set On Edge* is for you.

Third, if you have tried the conventional route and haven't gotten the results you've expected, and you're curious about trying another means of addressing your ACE-related health concerns, but not necessarily committed to an integrative approach, this book is not for you. I don't say this to be abrasive or off-putting; in fact, I actually have your best interest in mind when I say this. The fact is that the approach I am going to describe to you takes hard work and commitment, and if you're not fully committed to the approach, you likely will not get the results you're hoping to get. It may be in your best interest to postpone implementing the approach until you are able to put forth your best effort and be fully committed to it.

If you are committed to an integrative approach and want to do your best to obtain optimal health while reducing or avoiding your use of pharmaceutical medication, then this book is definitely for you. In my clinical practice, the women who achieve the best results when addressing their ACE-related chronic health concerns tend to be the ones who are most committed to an integrative approach and are willing to put in the hard work required to see the results they desire.

Now that you know who this book is and is not for, let's begin.

CHAPTER 1

MADE FOR TV

....

How ACEs found me before I was born and changed my life and family tree forever

It was two days before my 27th birthday. I had been away from my phone for the majority of the day. Instead, I spent the day relaxing and running errands with my husband and son. When we returned home that evening, I noticed that Facebook was notifying me of a message request. Someone with whom I wasn't connected was attempting to contact me. That was when I read the message:

"Hi, I'm your sister from Trinidad … My sister and I were searching for you all for a very long time. Sorry that it took so long to finally get in contact. Hoping to hear from you soon."

I froze. I wasn't sure what to do, so I told my husband about it and then reached out to my older brother. He confirmed that he had been contacted as well, and so had my sister.

I had believed all along that my father had children with other women during the 13 tumultuous years that he and my mother were married and living together, but for some reason, perhaps because, to date, he has never admitted to his infidelity, being contacted by one of his other children really shook me. I guess with advancements in the digital age and social media, I should have expected this day to come, but for some reason it caught me off guard.

I responded to her the following morning, asking questions and trying to sort out the details of my father's mysterious past. She was 26 years old, just like I was, and informed me that our father's other daughter, who had a different mother and was 27 at the time, also wanted to connect with me. I initially took the virtual encounter at face value, but after I had time to process everything that had happened, it hit me.

When I woke up on the morning of my birthday, I felt like my world was in shambles. I had the second worst birthday of my life, topped only by my 15th, when my 27-year-old favorite uncle passed away unexpectedly from an undiagnosed heart condition on the day before my birthday. I spent my 27th birthday (and several days, maybe even weeks afterward) in tears. Even when my husband and son took me to one of my favorite local restaurants to celebrate, it was difficult for me to be in the moment and not think about the fact that I was now in contact with my father's other children.

To explain why this encounter was so disrupting to my world, you need a bit of backstory. I'll explain.

I was born and partially raised on the beautiful island of Trinidad, in the Caribbean. I spent my first eight years of life there. By the time I was born, my mom had known about the infidelity that was taking place in her marriage for over a year and, over time, she began struggling with severe anxiety, depression, and panic attacks as a result.

In fact, I remember my grandmother coming over to sponge-bathe my occasionally bed-ridden mother and wash her hair using a bedpan, because she was so debilitated by her anxiety, depression, and panic attacks that she couldn't do much for herself. At times when my mother would stand up to go to the bathroom, her heart would start racing. She would start feeling nauseated, experience difficulty breathing, and be overcome by a feeling of intense panic. In those moments, she was absolutely certain that she would die, but she didn't. You see, my mom was a fighter.

Some of my earliest memories of Trinidad consist of me power-walking up the hill adjacent to our house alongside my brother, sister, and mom as we chanted, "I must, I must, I must improve my health." In spite of all of the emotional stressors that came my mom's way, she never stopped fighting. She was determined to do whatever it took to regain her physical, mental, spiritual, and social wellbeing, in spite of her stressful circumstances.

My mom fought until she was able to move to the United States and divorce my father, and although the path there was winding and obstacle-ridden, she was eventually able to overcome her anxiety, depression, and panic attacks and come off of all three of the psychotropic medications that she had been prescribed. Today, my mom does not take any psych meds.

My mom's experience actually led to me enrolling in naturopathic medical school, and after my four years there, I was able to help her support her mental wellness and promote a healthy stress response using integrative therapies. Today, I thank God that, in addition to not being on psychotropic medication, my mom no longer needs the natural therapies on a daily basis. Given the level of stress she is under, my mom's mental health is superb. She is able to handle the stress that comes her way in a healthy manner. She has a positive outlook and is happily remarried. I consider her to be a survivor.

Now that you understand my history, here's why my mom's experience is so important: Although she is doing well emotionally, her experience definitely impacted me. In fact, I can honestly say that my parents' relationship helped shape me into the person I am today. It has helped me become the compassionate and caring doctor that I am, but it has also had less-desirable effects.

You see, although I only lived with my biological father for my first eight years of life, my environment affected me.

Here's what I mean: I was only a year and a half when my little sister was born. My mom was dealing with a lot in her struggle with anxiety and depression at the time, so she had to make some important decisions regarding parenting. She decided that since I was a toddler now, I could begin drinking from a sippy-cup instead of a bottle, sleeping in a bed instead of my crib, walking by myself instead of being carried, etc. That way, she'd still be able to parent all three of her children and give the new baby the attention she needed.

Because I was so young, I couldn't understand why my mom was making all of these changes so suddenly and directing all of the attention that I felt I still needed towards this new baby. I felt incredibly sad and even replaced. I became extremely sensitive and cried very frequently during my childhood.

I remember sitting on my mom's dresser at age four, looking into the mirror. My mom was lying on her bed, still trying to manage her own mental health. My brother and sister were teasing me, and I remember shouting at them, "Do you all want me to kill myself?!"

My mom had no idea where I, as a four-year-old child, had learned the concept of suicide. She was so depressed that she had wished for death many times during her pregnancy with me, but to her knowledge she had never expressed those sentiments to me or in my presence. When I said that, she began to panic. What mother wouldn't if their four-year-old baby said something like that? She was so shocked and had no idea what to do, so she just shouted at me, "Don't ever let me hear you say that again!" Of course, I misinterpreted her concern for anger and again, I felt rejected and hurt.

As you can imagine, these types of situations (as well as a few other things I endured in early childhood) took a toll on me emotionally. From a very early age, I developed the false belief that people would not like me if they got to know me for who I truly was, and I believe this was a direct result of the emotional trauma I experienced.

I began to develop more introverted qualities and I became extremely anxious in social situations. For example, even though I did very well in school, the thought of raising my hand to answer a question led to a dramatic physiological response within my body. Whenever my teacher would ask a question that I knew the answer to, or God forbid that she should say a word (such as "genetics") that sounded like my name, my heart would begin racing. My voice would become shaky, and on some occasions, I would even start sweating. All of this happened in spite of the fact that I *knew* that I knew the correct answer! Imagine what would happen if the teacher called on me and I didn't know the answer …

My early environment continued to have a negative impact on my social relationships even into adulthood. In fact, before we were in a relationship, I remember my husband being the first person to suggest that some of the things I do, say, and possibly think may be a result of my relationship (or lack thereof) with my biological father. I remember arguing with him.

'How could my lack of a relationship with him be affecting me? It's not like I don't have a dad. Since I was 11 years old, I've had a wonderful step-father who has been more than a dad to me,' I thought to myself.

At the time, I saw it as a slap in my dad's face for me to admit that the things I had learned about men and fathers from him were not enough to negate the things I had learned about these topics from my biological father.

Around age 22 or 23, however, I started to see that my husband was right, and that whether I liked it or not, my past had significantly impacted my life. At that time, I made the decision to do everything within my power to counteract the effects of my traumatic past on my life. It was hard work and a continual process, but I persisted in making progress. After a while, I became confident that my traumatic childhood would not have a hold on me for much longer.

When my father's daughters contacted me via Facebook, that sort of changed. I honestly felt trapped. I felt like I would never be able to free myself from my traumatic past. For years, I had attempted to forget the messy details of my early life and address the symptoms of social and separation anxiety that I had dealt with as a result. And now, at 27 years of age, when I finally felt like I had healed sufficiently from my tumultuous upbringing, here it was again, rearing its ugly head. And the worst part was that the negative emotions that the situation evoked from me convinced me that, even after all of the work I had put into finding healing, I had not sufficiently healed. It took several months for me to process these emotions and come to terms with my new reality. It's still a journey, but one that I welcome because progress along this journey is so rewarding.

Now back to my story. When all of this happened, I had already become aware of the concept of adverse childhood experiences, or ACEs. About a year or two before my 27th birthday, I had started seeing connections between childhood trauma and different chronic conditions in my patients. This led me to start searching for a medical explanation. That was when I came across the concept of ACEs, and it all started to make sense.

I found out that ACEs, or highly stressful experiences during childhood, significantly increase our risk for four major categories of chronic disease: mental health concerns like anxiety and depression, hormonal or reproductive concerns like abnormal menstrual cycles and infertility, autoimmune diseases like lupus and rheumatoid arthritis, and metabolic concerns like diabetes, heart disease, and obesity.

CHAPTER 1 MADE FOR TV

When I first heard about ACEs, I made the decision to learn everything I could about them so I could better help my patients and break the cycle in my own life, for myself and my children.

My mission to wage war against the increased risk for chronic physical and mental health conditions that comes about as a result of ACEs was solidified one day after a conversation with my mom. During one of our discussions on the effects of childhood trauma, my mom told me that if she had understood prenatal and maternal influences and the fact that adverse childhood experiences increase the risk for mental and physical health concerns, she would've done things differently.

She would have done whatever it took to shield her children from exposure to the stressful environment in which we were raised during our early years and protect us from the increased risk that we now carry for numerous chronic health concerns.

When I heard my mom say, "I would've done whatever it took," it had an effect on me. You see, whenever my mom determines to do something, she does it. Just like she made up her mind to regain her health after her initial setback and accomplished it, I knew that the words my mom was saying were true. If she had realized the effect that our environment would have on us, as her children, she would have done things differently.

That was the moment I first realized that the reason I was learning about ACEs and had experienced them in my own life was bigger than my children and me. I realized that many women are like my mom, and if they only understood the effects of ACEs, they would do everything within their power to overcome their predispositions and provide a better environment and world for themselves and their children.

This is why I've made it my mission to educate and empower other women like me who have been affected by ACEs to break the cycle in their own lives, rise above their past and present circumstances, defy their predispositions, and live life on their own terms. I've found this to be possible. In this book, using my comprehensive B.A.L.A.N.C.E. Framework™, which was designed to help ACE survivors optimize their health and prevent or address mental health concerns, reproductive problems, autoimmune diseases, and metabolic concerns, I'll show you how.

CHAPTER 2

RECENTLY FOUND

....

The sneaky culprit behind more than 30 diseases that you weren't paying attention to until now

Imagine this with me: You're driving peacefully along a country road, admiring the beautiful scenery, when suddenly a car in the lane of oncoming traffic veers into your lane and is heading directly toward you. You instantly become more alert, your body tenses up, and you prepare yourself to make the next appropriate decisions and face what is to come.

In that moment, what you're feeling is a direct result of the interaction of and cooperation between two organ systems—the nervous system and endocrine or hormonal system. We refer to this physiological process as the beginning phase of your "fight-or-flight" or stress response.

Now let's shift gears a bit and imagine that you're a child between birth and age 17 and you're experiencing some adversity. It could be any number of things: your parents being separated or getting divorced; seeing your mother or another caretaker treated violently; a member of your household being incarcerated or addicted to the use of harmful substances; having a household member with depression or another mental health concern; feeling like you aren't loved or protected by your family; not always having the food, clothing, or other essentials that you need during your childhood; physical, emotional, or sexual abuse; experiencing the loss of a parent or sibling; growing up in foster care; experiencing chronic childhood illness; or some other adverse childhood experience, which we refer to as ACE.

Whatever the form of adversity, if you've experienced ACEs, you're likely to have developed, as a direct result, a hyperactive stress response. You know the way you feel when a car is headed at rapid speed toward you? I'm going to make a case that a miniature, less intense version of that is likely taking place in your body every single day.

Let me explain.

While some research suggests that exposure to ACEs at 16 and 17 years of age may still be problematic, we know for sure that when we experience ACEs before the age of 16, it directly causes physiological changes within our brains and bodies. The younger we are when we begin to experience these ACEs, the more drastic the changes tend to be. These changes come about as a result of alterations in one of the mechanisms that controls our stress response, specifically the hypothalamic-pituitary-adrenal (HPA) axis.

How Stress Works

To best understand how the stress response works, I want you to think of it as having two divisions or arms that work together to accomplish the needs of the body. The first arm of the stress response involves the musculoskeletal and sympathetic nervous systems and is most relevant when you are exposed to acute or short-term stressors, such as a car swerving into your lane. After the car returns to its lane and you realize that you're safe, the stress response terminates and your body returns to its normal state.

Here's a summary of the pertinent science behind this arm: When your stress response is initially activated, your sympathetic nervous system causes a hormone called epinephrine (also known as adrenaline) to be released from the medullae of the adrenal glands, which are located directly above your kidneys. This occurs within two to three minutes of you being exposed to the stressor. When epinephrine is released, it increases your heart rate, boosts your energy supplies, and raises your blood pressure. This effectively prepares your body to fight or flee. It prepares you to face what is to come if the stressor does not resolve. If the stressor does resolve—the car finds its way back to its own lane before causing a head-on collision—then the stress response is terminated and epinephrine and other hormone levels decrease until the body returns to its normal state.

The second arm of the stress response works hand-in-hand with the first arm and involves the hypothalamic-pituitary-adrenal axis, which I mentioned is commonly referred to as the HPA axis. This arm of the stress response comes into play after the acute stress response is activated and when the stressor that we're exposed to becomes chronic or long-term. This would be more like if the car that swerved into your lane actually did hit you, and then later on you developed a persistent fear of being harmed whenever you were driving or riding in a vehicle. Now, instead of you being acutely stressed because an oncoming car entered your lane, gave you a scare, and then returned to its own lane allowing your body time to return to a normal state, your fear of being harmed while in a vehicle persists beyond hours and days, to maybe even months and years. Now every time you are in a vehicle (and possibly even for hours after you've arrived at your destination, or even when you're just dreaming of being in a vehicle), you experience increased activation of the chronic arm of the stress response via the HPA axis.

Here are the details of how the chronic arm of the stress response works in harmony with the acute arm: As we've seen, the stress response is initially activated minutes after we're exposed to a stressor. The acute stress response is activated in part by the sympathetic nervous system, which causes epinephrine or adrenaline to be released from the medullae of the adrenal glands. When the stressor becomes chronic, the HPA axis becomes far more involved in the activation of the stress response than the sympathetic nervous system, and it causes cortisol and similar hormones to be released from the cortices of the adrenal glands.

Again, here's a simplified version of the science: In a domino-like effect, the HPA axis releases cortisol through very specific steps. First of all, a region of your brain called the hypothalamus sends hormonal messengers like corticotropin releasing hormone, also known as CRH, to the anterior pituitary gland, which is also located within the brain. The pituitary gland then sends a hormonal messenger called adrenocorticotropic hormone, or ACTH, to the cortices of the adrenal glands, causing them to release the steroid hormone cortisol.

Hopefully you're beginning to see that while epinephrine and cortisol are both involved in the stress response, they play different roles. Whereas epinephrine is secreted almost immediately and works in the short-term, cortisol is released over a longer period of time, usually for several hours after we initially come into contact with a stressor, and has many long-term effects on the body.

When the HPA axis causes an increase in cortisol levels, several things happen. Cortisol raises your blood sugar; manages how your body uses carbohydrates, fats, and proteins; and—take note of this—may also cause changes within other body systems. This is because it has the ability to alter by ramping up or shutting down a variety of physiological processes in order to effectively do its job. This includes your digestive, reproductive, immune, and other body systems.[1]

This attribute of cortisol is extremely important; it's crucial to your understanding of how adversity during childhood increases your risk for several chronic mental and physical health concerns throughout your lifetime.

We'll revisit this special characteristic of cortisol soon. For now, let's talk a bit more about cortisol's foundational characteristics.

The Stress Hormone That Isn't All Bad

First of all, I want you to understand two essential characteristics of cortisol:

#1. As a function of our HPA axes, our adrenal glands release cortisol both when we aren't experiencing

significant stress and when we're exposed to stressors. Think about it like breathing. Pay attention to how you're breathing right now. Under normal circumstances, we breathe in a very specific way. When we're exercising or afraid, however, the depth or rate of our breathing may increase beyond what is considered normal for a person at rest. In the same way, when our bodies are functioning as they should and there is minimal negative stress, cortisol levels peak just before we wake up in the morning and then decline throughout the day, but cortisol levels can also increase in response to chronic exposure to stressors.

#2. **Cortisol isn't all bad.** As we'll see, cortisol serves very important purposes within the body. We've already discussed the domino-like effect involving cortisol that takes place as a part of the process of stress response activation. As a review, a region of the brain called the hypothalamus causes the release of a hormone called CRH, which then causes the pituitary gland to release another hormone called ACTH. ACTH then stimulates the adrenal cortex to release cortisol, and the chronic stress response becomes fully activated. Therefore, in essence, the first crucial role that cortisol plays in the body is in the activation of the chronic stress response.

Without cortisol, we would not be able to effectively respond to and manage stress.

Now I want to tell you about another reason why cortisol isn't all bad and why we need the hormone in order for our bodies to function optimally. In order for me to explain this, I need you to think of hormones as keys and receptors on the cells within the body as locks. When you insert the correct key into a lock and turn it, something happens—the door unlocks. In the same way, when the HPA axis is activated and cortisol reaches a certain level or increases at a certain rate within the body, cortisol molecules act like keys and bind to receptors, or locks, in the hypothalamus and pituitary gland. The binding of cortisol to these receptors causes something to happen—the turning off of the secretion of CRH and ACTH, the two main hormones that initially caused cortisol secretion to ramp up in the first place.

In physiology, we classify this process as a negative feedback loop. As the first phase of negative feedback loops, a domino-like series of events takes place in order to arrive at a certain end result. In our case, this first phase involves the cascade of events we've discussed multiple times now involving CRH, ACTH, and cortisol, and the end result is an increase in cortisol levels. The second phase of negative feedback loops involves the end product of the final step in the domino chain serving as a catalyst to turn off the domino-like effect. In this case, the cortisol travels back to the hypothalamus and pituitary gland and turns off the secretion of CRH and ACTH. As the levels of CRH and ACTH decrease, less cortisol is secreted and the body returns to its normal state, which we refer to as homeostasis.[2]

As you can see from this explanation, cortisol also plays a crucial role in turning off the stress response.

Now, I shared the science behind these processes in detail because I want you to get one key point: Cortisol is not the enemy. In fact, we need cortisol in order to function optimally. Instead, the problem arises when, for one reason or another, cortisol is no longer able to effectively activate or terminate the stress response and either help the body deal with a stressor or bring the body back to its normal state after you're exposed to a stressor. This is what wreaks havoc on our bodies and increases our risk for various chronic conditions as ACE survivors.

How ACEs Change The Brain And Body

Now that you understand how your body activates its stress response and the role that cortisol plays in the body, let's take it a step further. We discussed the activation of the chronic arm of the stress response, which is controlled by the HPA axis, as being what would happen if you were to develop a chronic fear of driving or riding in vehicles after a car accident. If this were to actually happen to you, your stress response would be chronically activated whenever you got into a car and maybe even whenever you thought about getting into a car. Your body would release cortisol and other hormones in response to this activation of the chronic arm of the stress response.

Activation of the stress response in this situation is very similar to what occurs within the body in the case of adverse childhood experiences. Because it's the simplest to illustrate, let's take the case of physical abuse complicated by addiction as an example. Let's say a child has a father who is physically abusive whenever he is intoxicated. When he isn't drunk, the child's father seems to be a decent person to be around. The child comes home from school at about 4:15 p.m. and he knows that his father usually comes home around 7:45 p.m. Because he has no way of knowing whether or not his father has been drinking (and ultimately what his own night will be like) until he gets home, the child develops a chronic fear of being at home when his father comes home.

This psychological fear leads to activation of the stress response and the child's adrenal cortices churn out cortisol in response to the HPA axis' direction. This prepares him to face this chronic, persistent stressor. As long as his father continues to drink and be physically abusive to him while intoxicated, and as long as he continues to live in the home where he is exposed to this stressor, the stressor persists and his stress response remains chronically activated.

Now I want to make it clear that ACEs are slightly different from the scenario we described earlier involving the fear of another car accident, and I'll explain why. Here's a hint: It has to do with our age and the development of our brains when we're first exposed to these chronic stressors.

When we experience adverse events, specifically during childhood, it has long-lasting effects on our brains and bodies. Chronic stress, and especially chronic childhood stress, literally changes our physiology and can even change the way our brains are wired.

Here's how: Because the structures of the brain are still being developed during childhood and are vulnerable to change at this time, excessive activation of the stress response during this early developmental period can reprogram the HPA axis and lead to changes in other structures of the brain's limbic system.

Because of this reprogramming, people who have experienced early life stress tend to have altered HPA-axis activity as adults, both at baseline, which we consider to be their "normal," and during acute and chronic stress.[3] This is regardless of whether or not they continued to experience high stress after the age of 18, when their HPA axes were far more developed.[4]

Early life stress can change the HPA axis in one of two ways. First of all, ACE-induced reprogramming of the HPA axis can result in hypoactivity of the HPA axis. This is where the body loses its ability to react to stressors and you begin to have a difficult time mounting a stress response. Second, ACE-induced reprogramming of the HPA axis can result in hyperactivity, where your brain and body sort of get used to high levels of cortisol and set your "normal" at a higher state of stress response activation. This causes the body to have an exaggerated response when you're exposed to stressors.

Let's explore these concepts.

HPA-Axis Hypoactivity-
True HPA-axis hypoactivity is the less common of the two findings in affected ACE survivors. It comes about after we've been hyperfunctioning for some time, and we tend to see this hypoactivity in individuals who have been diagnosed with post-traumatic stress disorder, or PTSD, as a result of the things they experienced in their childhood. Essentially what happens in these cases is that the stress response is repeatedly activated in the early phases of trauma exposure and CRH increases to abnormally high levels. This leads to something else happening within the body. I'll explain.

You now know that as a part of the domino-like effect we've discussed, the increase in CRH is supposed to lead to an increase in ACTH, which leads to an increase in cortisol, but it doesn't happen this way for these people. I'm going to tell you what actually happens with these people, but if you don't understand at first, just stick with me. I'm also going to use a similar analogy to the one we used earlier to explain what I mean. In our discussion on cortisol earlier, we talked about hormones as keys and receptors as locks. Like cortisol, CRH is a hormone, so after I tell you what happens, I'm going to use the same analogy to make the concept clearer.

Now that you know exactly what to expect, here's what actually happens: In response to the chronically activated stress response and the high CRH levels, and in an attempt to modulate the stress response, these people's bodies actually decrease the expression of CRH receptors at the level of the pituitary gland.

Here's what that means: You'll remember that, under normal circumstances, the hormone or key, CRH, typically binds to receptors, which we're thinking of as locks, at the level of the pituitary gland in order to increase ACTH, which then increases cortisol levels. Well, I want you to think about what's happening specifically in these people's brains as though this process started to occur, but CRH was unlocking the door too often, so the brain just decided to remove most of the locks that fit the CRH key from the doors at the level of the pituitary gland.

With fewer CRH receptors present, these individuals' CRH is less able to stimulate the release of ACTH and their cortisol levels do not rise as much as they had in the past in response to elevated CRH levels. Essentially, the body attempts to compensate for the initial hyperactivation of the HPA axis by decreasing CRH receptors at the pituitary gland. This results in hypofunctioning of the HPA axis. Because there aren't as many locks, their bodies no longer respond to CRH as they should, and because their cortisol levels no longer rise as much as they had in the past, these individuals tend to have a difficult time mounting an appropriate stress response as adults, even when they're exposed to significant stressors.

HPA-Axis Hyperactivity-

Hyperactivity of the HPA axis, on the other hand, which is the most common finding in adults who have been affected by ACEs, essentially results in your body having an exaggerated response to stressors of all kinds. Individuals with hyperactive HPA axes tend to have higher CRH levels and higher daytime levels of cortisol.[5]

We've discussed cortisol's role in both activating and terminating the stress response, but cortisol also plays another significant role as it pertains to the immune system. This role is especially important to our understanding of how ACE-induced hyperactivity of the HPA axis increases our risk for several chronic diseases. Do you remember our discussion about cortisol's special ability to alter other bodily functions, including the immune system, in order to accomplish its job? Well, it has a lot to do with that.

Here's a bit more of the story: Under normal circumstances, activation of the stress response results in immune system changes. When we're exposed to an acute stressor, inflammation levels initially increase. As the stress progresses and becomes chronic, cortisol is released and higher levels suppress various aspects of the immune system. As cortisol levels continue to rise, the hormone normally binds to receptors on various cells within the body in order to decrease the immune response. This process is similar to the way that cortisol travels back to the hypothalamus and pituitary gland where it decreases CRH and ACTH production in order to help decrease cortisol levels and restore balance. Essentially, under normal circumstances, cortisol terminates both the immune response and the stress response in order to help the body return to its normal state after HPA-axis activation.

In people who have developed hyperactive HPA axes as a result of ACE exposure, however, again, it doesn't exactly happen this way. Despite having high cortisol levels, these people tend to have a hard time terminating the immune response and stress response. We believe this is due to problems with cortisol's ability to bind to the receptors in order to bring about the necessary changes. We refer to this binding capability as cortisol signaling. Problems with cortisol signaling impair the hormone's ability to efficiently bind to receptors on cells in order to modulate the immune system, as well as to bind to cells in the hypothalamus and pituitary gland in order to terminate the stress response via the negative feedback loop we discussed.

This problem impairs cortisol's ability to shut down both the immune response and the stress response in order to help the body return to its normal state. It also contributes to an unrestrained inflammatory state within the body and increases our risk for a variety of chronic physical and mental health concerns in adulthood.[6] Essentially, people with hyperactive stress responses as a result of the ACEs they've experienced in early life tend to have high levels of cortisol, but due to problems with cortisol signaling, they have a difficult time turning off their stress and immune responses; their stress responses remain in a state of constant activation, and their immune responses go haywire, increasing their risk for multiple inflammatory and otherwise chronic diseases.

Why Did I Share That?

There's a reason why I went into such great detail explaining how ACEs impact our HPA axes and our lives in general. My aim in sharing this information with you is to explain the physiology behind how ACEs affect us—specifically how your past experiences could be affecting your current state of health. I often encounter people who have experienced ACEs and, as a result of their subsequent physical and mental health concerns, report being told by others to "just act normal," "just try to be happy," or the classic "but you don't look sick."

Hearing these things over and over again takes a toll on them and they begin to believe that they may actually be the problem, that if they could just "act more normal," their lives would be easier. They begin to erroneously blame themselves for what they're experiencing and for what they view as their shortcomings.

I've found that, when we understand that our increased risk for these health concerns and related complications is the natural result of physiological changes that have taken place within our brains and bodies as a result of our childhood environments, we are far more able to be patient with ourselves and to view ourselves as we truly are—survivors of adverse childhood experiences.

We're able to celebrate our victories instead of focusing on what we perceive to be our shortcomings. I hope that, if you've had negative self-talk or been adversely affected by the expressed opinions of others, these explanations will have this effect for you and help you to be more accepting of who you are and of the circumstances that you've been able to overcome so far in life.

ACEs literally touch every area of our lives, but the positive news is that research shows that by taking measures to stabilize the HPA axis, addressing brain changes, decreasing inflammation, and, of course, addressing the residual emotional, physiological, and other effects of the trauma, we can effectively decrease our health risk, become the best version of ourselves, and live the lives we were truly created to live.

CHAPTER 3

MYTH-BUSTER

....

The two most damaging myths that frustrate effective treatment, waste time and energy, and drain your emotions

BEFORE WE GO ANY further, I want to share some common myths regarding ACEs. I believe it's important for me to share these widespread but erroneous beliefs because neglecting to share them could mean that I am helping to perpetuate these extremely damaging misconceptions.

The "That Doesn't Happen In Families Like Ours" Myth

One of the most common misconceptions when it comes to this topic is the false belief that ACEs happen to a certain type of people. I've made it my business to do everything within my power to debunk this damaging idea.

I still remember when it first occurred to me that this may be an issue. I was in the middle of an appointment with a patient when she shared a few new details about the insomnia she had been experiencing over the previous six or so years. These details suggested that she may have been experiencing HPA-axis dysregulation, so I started to talk with her about ACEs.

I asked the patient if she had ever heard the term "adverse childhood experiences" and she said no, so I proceeded to explain the concept. Next, I shared a few of the most common examples, including parents being separated or divorced, substance abuse in the household, and not feeling loved or protected by family. Then I asked her if she had experienced anything like that growing up. When I asked this question, she started to stutter, became visibly uncomfortable, and then mumbled something to the effect of, "Yeah, I think I've experienced some of those things."

CHAPTER 3 MYTH-BUSTER

As soon as I noticed her discomfort, I began to suspect that she may have held an incorrect underlying belief about the type of people who experience ACEs. I figured that perhaps she thought ACEs happened to people of a certain education level, race, ethnicity, or socioeconomic status. I took a few minutes to educate her about how common ACEs are and why there is no need to be embarrassed or ashamed about having experienced them. After my explanation, she relaxed again and we continued with our appointment. Although I had just started learning about ACEs at that time, it was at this moment that I made a mental note to do everything I could to debunk this damaging belief that is not founded upon reality and that has the potential to prevent people from seeking and receiving the medical help they need.

Since that encounter, I've had other people suggest this idea to me without really coming out and stating that this was their underlying belief. I've even had patients who were more direct in their approach tell me that ACEs don't happen in families like theirs. These patients honestly believed that what they were telling me was true, but that didn't make their beliefs factual.

Here are the facts: First of all, the original ACE study was conducted on middle-class, mostly college-educated people in the Kaiser Health group, 74.8% of which were Caucasian. The fact that they were in the Kaiser Health Group indicates that they had steady jobs or some other reliable means of paying for health insurance. About two out of three individuals within this group of people—63.9%, to be precise—had experienced at least one ACE.[7]

Furthermore, the World Health Organization's World Mental Health Surveys estimate that across all countries, regardless of how economically developed they are, around 40% of people have experienced at least one ACE.[8]

So let's clear this misconception up once and for all. Here's what it boils down to: It's the nature of statistics that the percentage of people in your sample who have experienced ACEs will change depending on who you include in the study. It's also true that you could conceivably manipulate the results of your study by carefully selecting the people you interview or the questions that you ask.

For example, while each class of people may have ACEs that are more common among them (and you could certainly make it appear as though ACEs only occur among a certain class of people if you only interview certain classes of people or if you only ask about the ACEs that are most common among a specific class), the truth is that if we look at all ACEs as a general category of life events, we'll find that they are common among all people groups and across all socioeconomic statuses.

In other words, if you look at a wide variety of reliable ACE research and survey results, you'll find that while certain ACEs may be more common among certain classes of people, the number of people who have experienced any ACE, regardless of demographics, tends to fall between 40 and 60 percent.

The truth is that ACEs are common across all income levels, races, ethnicities, and cultures, and we need to change the conversation surrounding ACEs so that we, as survivors, can receive the trauma-informed care that we need in order to break the cycle and live our healthiest and best lives now.

The "I Don't Need To Tell My Doctor" Myth

Now that brings us to the next most common misconception that I hear regarding ACEs, and that is the belief that the treatment for the health conditions that we are at increased risk for as ACE survivors will not change, so we don't need to disclose our trauma history to our healthcare providers or seek care from specialized, trauma-informed healthcare professionals.

I believe that this very damaging belief is the result of a misunderstanding concerning the difference between treatment goals and treatment options. Treatment goals are the outcomes or results that we hope to accomplish, while treatment options are the specific therapies or treatments that we use to accomplish our overarching goals. As ACE survivors, our treatment goals are mostly the same as non-ACE survivors, but the treatment options we select may vary.

Here's an example: If you're diagnosed with type-2 diabetes as an ACE survivor, our treatment goals are going to be the same as our treatment goals for any non-ACE survivor with type-2 diabetes—decrease blood sugar, improve insulin sensitivity, prevent complications like end-organ damage and diabetic ulcers, and maintain or improve quality of life. Our treatment options, on the other hand, specifically the way we arrive at our treatment goals, may, or at least should, vary.

One explanation of why treatment options should vary for ACE survivors compared to their non-ACE-surviving counterparts is that ACE survivors have increased risks for some co-morbidities or co-occurring disorders. Let's look at a specific example: Insulin is a hormone that helps keep our blood sugar within the normal range. It does this by helping glucose molecules leave our bloodstream and go into our cells where they can be used to produce energy. People who have been diagnosed with type-2 diabetes have some degree of insulin resistance, which is a condition in which the insulin needed to regulate blood sugar is present within the body, but the body has become less responsive to it. Insulin resistance causes the elevated blood sugar that we see in type-2 diabetes.

Many people aren't aware of the fact that, in addition to regulating blood sugar, insulin also plays a significant role in regulating the HPA axis. In cases of insulin resistance or type-2 diabetes, where the body becomes less responsive to insulin, not only is insulin less able to regulate blood sugar, but it is also less able to do its job in regulating the HPA axis. This results in people with insulin resistance and/or diabetes being at increased risk for depression.[9]

This is across the board for all people with type-2 diabetes, but in many cases, there are other protective factors at play that prevent people with diabetes from becoming depressed. Therefore, we don't see this increased risk for depression develop into an actual diagnosis of a depressive disorder in every case.

In the specific case of a person with type-2 diabetes who I know has experienced ACEs and is likely to have already developed a dysregulated HPA axis as a result, however, this information is almost always highly relevant. The dysregulation of the HPA axis that comes about as a result of insulin resistance is oftentimes enough to push an ACE survivor whose HPA-axis function is already abnormal over the edge and into a depressed state. Keeping this in mind, I tailor my ACE-surviving patients' treatment plans to meet their individual needs.

Here's how: When selecting therapeutic agents to help accomplish our treatment goals for my patients' diabetes, I tend to start with minimally invasive treatment options with low to non-existent side-effect profiles that help decrease their blood sugar and increase their bodies' sensitivity to insulin. This is where the treatment options vary. Out of the many therapies that can help us achieve our treatment goals, unless there is a contraindication such as a medication interaction or an allergy, for my ACE survivors, I select the ones that help us achieve our treatment goals of improved glycemic control and that also have a regulatory or otherwise positive effect on the HPA axis.

Essentially, knowing that they have had traumatic pasts and are predisposed to HPA-axis dysregulation (and that, as a result, they are at a much higher risk for depression than both non-diabetic ACE survivors and people with diabetes who have not experienced ACEs), I support their HPA-axis function in order to decrease the likelihood of them becoming depressed or the likelihood of their depression worsening if they've previously been diagnosed with a depressive disorder. Now the conversation is no longer "take this metformin (or cinnamon or insert-any-therapy-here) for your diabetes because this is where we start," but instead it becomes "what is the best treatment option for your diabetes given your trauma history and other pertinent health history?"

Here's a more specific example: For my ACE survivors who have been diagnosed with diabetes, I usually put together an individualized, herbal, hypoglycemic formula. When I select my hypoglycemic herbs for ACE survivors, instead of only choosing herbs that are purely hypoglycemic or insulin-sensitizing in nature, I include herbs such as Ashwagandha (*Withania somnifera*) that have been shown in pre-clinical studies to decrease blood sugar and enhance the body's insulin sensitivity[10-11] and are also adaptogenic in nature and have been shown to help regulate the HPA axis and normalize cortisol levels in humans.[12]

Because I am aware of the effects of childhood trauma on the physical and mental health conditions that I treat and on quality of life in general, I always ask my patients about their trauma histories. You may be seeing a practitioner who is also aware of these effects and is able to individualize your treatment options to address your increased risk as an ACE survivor, but if your provider is not aware of your ACE status, he or she may assume that you have an ACE score of zero and may not individualize your treatment plan to address all aspects of your health as a result.

Here's another example of how treatment options can change and why you should share the fact that you have experienced ACEs with your healthcare providers: The results of many studies support the idea that depression may be inflammatory in nature. Most of the researchers arrived at this conclusion by conducting randomized, controlled clinical trials in which they took a group of people with depression and randomly divided them into two groups. They gave one group an anti-inflammatory therapy, which ranged in different studies from fish oil to aspirin, and they gave the other group a placebo or sugar pill. At the end of the studies I'm describing, researchers found that the group that was given the anti-inflammatory therapy experienced improvements in their depression, while the placebo group did not. This led them to conclude that depression may be caused by an inflammatory state, and this is why therapies that reduced inflammation also led to a reduction in symptoms of depression. That's simple and straightforward enough.

Here's the catch. Other groups of researchers came forward afterward attempting to replicate the studies. Some of them found similar results, but others were unable to demonstrate that anti-inflammatory therapies led to any improvement in depressive symptoms;

they found little difference between the symptoms of the anti-inflammatory group and the placebo group at the end of their studies. As you can imagine, this led to a lot of confusion. Why would anti-inflammatory therapies help in some people and make very little difference in others? No one could find the answer until a group of researchers decided to divide a group of individuals up in a different way to study them.

In November 2018, a study was published in which researchers divided a group of people into three groups—people diagnosed with major depressive disorder (MDD) who had experienced ACEs, people with MDD who had not experienced ACEs, and a control group of healthy volunteers who had not experienced ACEs.[13] When they tested their inflammatory markers, the group of ACE survivors who were diagnosed with MDD showed higher levels of inflammation than both their non-ACE-surviving counterparts with depression and the healthy control group.

The results of this study were monumental, in my opinion, because they provided a potential explanation for why some people's depression may have responded to anti-inflammatory therapies while others' did not. If your inflammatory markers are already within the normal range, then we would not expect much of a change in any inflammation-based health condition from taking anti-inflammatory therapies, but on the other hand, if your inflammatory markers are abnormal and you take anti-inflammatory therapies, we would expect to see a reduction in your inflammatory markers and an improvement in any health condition that was caused or worsened by your previously high levels of inflammation.

The researchers' study led them to draw what appears to be a more accurate conclusion than the black-and-white studies I described previously that sought to answer the question, "Is depression an inflammatory illness or not?" Instead, the researchers in this study concluded that there is likely a subtype of depression that is responsive to anti-inflammatory therapies, and as a result of the changes that take place with the HPA axis, immune system, and vagus nerve when we experience childhood trauma, this subtype is more commonly seen in individuals who have experienced ACEs. Therefore, using anti-inflammatory therapies to address depression is most likely to be beneficial in ACE survivors compared to their non-ACE-surviving counterparts.

This is just another illustration of the fact that sharing your trauma history with your medical providers or selecting providers who are knowledgeable concerning the effects of ACEs can make a difference in your treatment plan. It can be the difference between whether a therapy will be very effective for you or whether it will have little effect at all, and as a result, it can significantly affect the quality of the results you see on your current treatment plan.

Hopefully these examples have either strengthened your belief or opened your eyes to the fact that treatment options can (and should) vary between ACE survivors and their non-ACE-surviving counterparts, even when they are diagnosed with the same health conditions, because individualizing the treatment to one's health history leads to the most comprehensive and, in my experience, effective care.

CHAPTER 4

BRAIN STRAIN

....

How ACEs change your brain and create a breeding ground for mental health concerns in later life

As we've discussed, experiencing traumatic events during childhood can literally change our brains. So far, we've discussed the changes that can occur as it relates to the HPA axis, and now we'll discuss a few other key changes that can take place within the brains of ACE survivors.

Brain Changes In ACE-Surviving Children And Adults

To study these changes, researchers followed three groups of children in Romania—one group that was raised in a loving home environment with biological parents, one group that had been raised within an institution for abandoned children, and one group that was raised in an institution and then transferred to a high-quality fostering arrangement.[14]

Before we proceed, I want to be clear that the children who were institutionalized experienced severe, early emotional and physical neglect, both of which we've identified as ACEs. While in these institutions, they received regimented care and were largely deprived of the physical and emotional interaction that children typically receive when growing up in a household with loving adults who are invested in their future wellbeing.

Now that we've made that clear, let's continue. After randomly assigning institutionalized children to either remain in the institution or be rerouted to foster care, researchers began to conduct imaging studies, including magnetic resonance imaging studies (MRIs) and electroencephalograms (EEGs), in order to evaluate the structure and function of their brains. They wanted to compare their brain structures before reassignment to their brains after reassignment, as well as to those of children who were developing normally.

The results of these studies were fascinating. Researchers found that both the group of children who had previously been institutionalized and the group that was still institutionalized at the time of the imaging studies had smaller volumes of gray matter in their cerebral cortices compared to the healthy controls. When it came to the white matter, however, the group that was still institutionalized at the time of the study and was not sent to an improved foster care environment had significantly smaller amounts of cortical white matter compared to the group that was previously but no longer institutionalized and the group that was never institutionalized.

The Basics Of Gray- And White-Matter Development

To understand the principles that may potentially be underlying the results of this and similar studies, you'll need to understand how the gray and white matter in our brains develop. First of all, I want you to think of gray matter as being associated with various skills and abilities and white matter as what determines how quickly we process information. When it comes to gray matter, we are born with a certain amount, and this typically increases until puberty, at which point communication between brain cells becomes more efficient and the brain begins to eliminate less efficient communication pathways. Through this process, which is referred to as neural pruning, we begin to see a decline in gray matter starting around puberty. White matter, on the other hand, is pretty straightforward; as we grow older, the amount of white matter we have tends to increase.

ACEs And Gray Matter

Here is the significance of this background information in connection with the results of the study I've shared: The fact that the children who had previously been institutionalized and those who were presently institutionalized at the time the study was conducted had smaller amounts of gray matter in their brains than those who had never been institutionalized is likely a result of one of two things. The first option is that this could represent a deficit, where the children simply developed less gray matter than their peers did. The second option is that the study results could actually represent an acceleration in development.

For example, we've discussed the fact that the normal developmental trend is for gray matter to increase until puberty and then, through neural pruning, decrease for the duration of the lifespan. Based on this fact, the underlying reason for the study results we see could be that the neglect that the children who had been institutionalized experienced led to them developing less gray matter than is typical in early life.

On the other hand, it could also be that the institutionalized children matured faster, in a sense, and experienced the neural pruning we discussed at an accelerated rate compared to their never-institutionalized peers. In other words, their brains started the process of destroying connections and communication pathways that appeared to be redundant or less useful at a much earlier age than is typical.

While it may seem beneficial, this process is problematic because the brains of young children simply don't have the experience necessary to determine which connections are important and which are dispensable. Their brains may conduct neural pruning based on their negative experiences early in life instead of based on positive experiences as is typical of pruning that occurs in adolescence.

While we don't currently have the research we need to definitively determine which of the two hypotheses that I've shared is the underlying cause of institutionalized children having lower volumes of gray matter, the results are clear. Gray matter volume is associated with intellectual ability[15] and skills such as emotional control and processing.[16] As a result, having lower quantities of gray matter in early life changes the typical course of brain development and makes children more vulnerable to problems later in life.

Speaking in very general terms, children with lower quantities of gray matter tend to have lower IQs and more problems with controlling and processing their emotions than they would have if they had larger volumes of gray matter.

Fortunately, however, this isn't the end of the story. Even for adult ACE survivors whose childhood experiences have increased the likelihood of us having smaller volumes of gray matter than we may have had if our experiences had been different, there is hope. When we talk about the B.A.L.A.N.C.E. Framework™, I'll share some interventions that have been shown to increase cortical gray matter and therefore improve outcomes like emotional control and processing.

ACEs And White Matter

When it comes to white matter, we only have one hypothesis that attempts to explain the changes we see in children who have survived ACEs. Here it is: The fact that children who were institutionalized at the time that the study was conducted had smaller volumes of white matter than both children who had never been institutionalized and those who had previously been institutionalized may represent a developmental delay. We suspect that white matter may be increasing at a slower pace in these individuals.

The results of this study demonstrate, however, that white matter volume can improve when children who have survived ACEs are removed from their stressful or otherwise negative environments. The fact that the group that was previously but no longer institutionalized at the time of the study showed similar white matter volumes to the group that was never institutionalized is great news! It suggests that children who have survived ACEs may have the opportunity to "catch up" where white matter is concerned in adolescence or even adulthood.

ACEs And Mental Health Risk

As we've discussed, experiencing childhood adversity can significantly alter brain function and development and increase our risk for various mental health concerns as a result. So far, we have research that demonstrates a correlation between ACEs and depressive disorders (including major depression, persistent depressive disorder),[17] anxiety spectrum disorders (including generalized anxiety disorder, social phobia, and panic disorder),[18-19] bipolar disorder,[19-20] post-traumatic stress disorder,[18-19] substance abuse disorders,[19] hallucinations, schizophrenia and other forms of psychosis,[21] and attempted suicide.[22]

Here are a few of the available statistics from various studies:

- Exposure to ACEs is associated with increased risk of depressive disorders up to decades after their occurrence.[17] One study demonstrated that individuals who had experienced one or more ACE were at increased risk for experiencing depressive symptoms later in life, and the degree of risk was contingent upon the level of social support they had. For example, those with more than one ACE who reported limited social support had almost a threefold increase in depressive symptoms later in life, compared to those with limited social support who had experienced no ACEs. Among those with moderate social support, ACE survivors were 2.21 times more likely to develop depressive symptoms than non-ACE survivors were, and among those with strong social support, ACE survivors were 1.39 times more likely to develop depressive symptoms than non-ACE survivors were.[24]

- Individuals who had experienced four or more categories of childhood exposure, compared to those who had experienced none, had fourfold to twelvefold increased health risks for alcoholism, drug abuse, depression, and suicide attempts, and a twofold to fourfold increase in smoking.[22]

- Compared to individuals who did not report any sexual abuse, ACE-surviving men and women who reported a history of childhood sexual abuse were more than twice as likely to have attempted suicide. Compared with those who did not report childhood sexual abuse, men and women exposed to childhood sexual abuse were at a 40% increased risk of marrying an alcoholic, and a 40% to 50%

increased risk of reporting current problems with their marriages.[25]

- Compared to individuals who did not experience any ACEs, the risks of heavy drinking, self-reported alcoholism, and marrying an alcoholic were increased twofold to fourfold in individuals with multiple ACEs, regardless of whether or not their parents had problems with alcohol.[26]

- Compared with individuals who did not experience any ACEs, people who experienced five or more ACEs were seven to ten times more likely to report using illicit drugs, being addicted to illicit drugs, and intravenous drug use. In these individuals, each additional ACE increased the likelihood of starting to use illicit drugs at an earlier age twofold to fourfold.[27]

- Compared to people with no ACEs, people with seven or more ACEs were 500% more likely to report experiencing hallucinations. The hallucinations reported in this study were not due to substance use.[28]

ACE Survivors And Psychotropic Medication

To add to the complexity of this situation, individuals with an ACE score of 5 or more were nearly three times as likely to be prescribed psychotropic medication, compared to those who were not exposed to any traumatic events during childhood.[29]

The increased likelihood of ACE survivors being prescribed these medications varied by the type of drug. When we break it down by drug classes, we find that people with ACE scores of 5 or more were three times more likely to be prescribed antidepressants, two times more likely to be prescribed anti-anxiety medication, ten times more likely to be prescribed antipsychotics, and 17 times more likely to be prescribed mood stabilizers than people with ACE scores of zero.

You may think, 'Well, this makes sense.' If we have an increased risk for mental health concerns, then of course we'll be more likely to be prescribed medication for these concerns. However, it's important for us to keep three facts in mind as we process this information:

Fact #1: According to the National Institute of Mental Health, one out of three people with depressive disorders will not experience remission from their mental health concerns, even after trying up to four different antidepressants.[30] In other words, for at least 33% of people, drugs will not solve the problem. While this statistic pertains specifically to antidepressants, the same can be said for all classes of psychotropic medication; they don't always bring about the desired results.

Fact #2: For the people who are able to effectively address their mental health concerns using psychotropic medication, these benefits may come with unwanted effects. For example, many (though not all) psychotropic drugs are unsafe during pregnancy and breastfeeding, so women may find themselves having to choose between their own mental health and the health of their unborn or soon-to-be-born children if psychotropic medication is their only method of addressing their mental health.

Furthermore, antidepressant use during pregnancy has been associated with increased risk of pregnancy-induced hypertension, with or without pre-eclampsia in mothers,[31] and some research suggests that antidepressant use during pregnancy may be associated with increased risk for autism spectrum disorders and psychiatric conditions (e.g. depressive disorders, bipolar disorder, anxiety spectrum disorders, attention-deficit and attention-deficit hyperactivity disorder, conduct disorder, schizophrenia, etc.) in offspring, compared to the children of mothers who were never prescribed psychotropic medication or who discontinued their medication prior to pregnancy. In this particular study, the children of mothers who had never been prescribed psychotropic medication prior to pregnancy but who started taking the drugs while pregnant had the greatest incidence of psychiatric disorders.[32]

My purpose in sharing this research is not to guilt any expecting mothers into weaning off of their medication. Just as there are risks associated with taking psychotropic medication during pregnancy, there are risks associated with having untreated psychiatric concerns during pregnancy. If you need the medication to keep yourself and your child safe, it's the best thing you can do, and this does not make you any less of a mother or woman. I simply want to share this information so that women who are not currently pregnant but may or would like to become pregnant and who are taking or considering taking psychotropic medication can consider these facts and make more informed choices, such as seeking out ways to address their mental health concerns without the use of medication before they get pregnant.

The unwanted effects of psychotropic medication are also relevant to those of us who have decided against or are finished having children. This is because many psychotropic medications, including very common ones like antidepressants[33] and antipsychotics,[34] increase the rate of metabolic concerns such as diabetes, cardiovascular disease, and obesity. When we couple this fact with the fact that, as ACE survivors, we are already at increased risk for these metabolic concerns, we can see that we have a potentially problematic situation on our hands.

Fact #3: Psychotropic medication is not the only way to address mental health concerns. In my opinion, it is not the best way to address mental health concerns in most cases, and in the vast majority of cases, psychotropic medication should be used as a final resort when it comes to improving our mental health, especially as women who have survived ACEs.

My all-time favorite quote from the Journal of Addiction Medicine puts it very eloquently, and while they're talking specifically about anxiety and benzodiazepines, this principle can be applied to most if not all cases of mental health concerns. "Anxiety is not a benzodiazepine-deficiency disease. It is possible to treat anxiety

CHAPTER 4 BRAIN STRAIN

and insomnia without medicines of any kind, and it is possible to use medicines other than benzodiazepines for these common and serious mental disorders."[35]

With my patients in my clinical practice, I've been privileged to see that there is a better way to address mental health concerns and the other effects of the traumatic childhood events that predispose us to these concerns. By uncovering and addressing the multi-pronged causes of these health concerns, we can see big shifts in our lives, and I'll show you how this can be your experience when we talk about my B.A.L.A.N.C.E. Framework™ for optimizing physical and mental health in ACE survivors.

CHAPTER 5

FEMALE PARTS

....

How ACEs increase risk for female health issues, reduce fertility, and keep you from enjoying the family you always pictured

Do you remember a time when you were under a lot of psychological or even physical stress, so much so that it altered your normal menstrual cycle? Maybe your period came early or late, or maybe it didn't come at all that month. We've known for many years that high levels of acute stress can negatively influence reproductive function, but a growing body of research is now demonstrating that chronic stress, and particularly chronic childhood stress, can lead to menstrual irregularities and impaired fertility.

Here's how: We know that childhood stress disrupts the normal function of the hypothalamus and pituitary gland and, if unchecked, leads to HPA-axis hyperactivity. This is relevant to reproductive function because many of the hormones involved in HPA-axis function actually inhibit hormones that are essential for the optimal function of the reproductive system.

To more fully understand how the HPA axis and reproductive system interact, let's take a second look at the hypothalamus and pituitary gland. We've discussed the hypothalamus as being a region of the brain that controls various nervous system and hormonal functions, among other things. We also mentioned that, as a function of the HPA axis, the hypothalamus releases corticotropin-releasing hormone, or CRH, which then acts on the pituitary gland.

CRH is not the only hormone that the hypothalamus secretes; it also secretes other releasing hormones, with the most pertinent one to our discussion on ACEs and reproductive health being gonadotropin-releasing hormone, or GnRH. When GnRH is released by the hypothalamus, it travels to and acts upon the pituitary gland. Similar to what happens with the HPA axis, this releasing hormone causes the pituitary gland to release hormones. In this case, the hormones are called luteinizing hormone (LH) and follicle-stimulating hormone (FSH). In women, LH and FSH then act upon our ovaries to increase the production of the hormones we most readily associate with reproduction, such as estrogen and progesterone. This process is referred to as the hypothalamic-pituitary-gonadal, or HPG, axis.

Here we see two parallel axes, the HPA axis and HPG axis, which have important and complex effects on each other. For example, the HPA-axis hormone CRH inhibits the HPG axis hormone GnRH, so that when CRH levels are high, such as in the case of trauma-induced HPA-axis hyperactivation, GnRH levels are low.[36] When GnRH levels are low, LH and FSH levels are also low, and we see abnormalities in our other hormone levels like estrogen and progesterone as well. In women, low LH and FSH levels are associated with irregular or absent menstrual cycles and infertility. Furthermore, cortisol inhibits LH, estrogen, and progesterone, so that these levels are low when cortisol levels are high, and the relationships that exist between these two axes are even further complicated by the fact that some reproductive hormones, such as estrogen, actually stimulate the genes that control our HPA-axis hormones.[36]

ACEs And Reproductive Disorder Risk

As is the case with all of the correlations that researchers note between ACEs and chronic disease risk, being a part of a statistical group that shares increased risk for certain conditions does not mean that you will be diagnosed with or meet the criteria for every single condition; it simply means that you are more likely to meet these conditions than you would be if you had not experienced ACEs. Now that we've gotten that cleared up, I'll share what the research shows about the correlation between ACEs and reproductive health concerns.

So far, the research demonstrates that, as a statistical group compared to women who have not experienced childhood adversity, women who have experienced ACEs are more likely to experience shorter gestational age (e.g. ACE-surviving women are more likely to have their babies prior to 40 weeks) and lower birth weight;[37] more likely to be engaged in risky health behaviors, including smoking, alcohol use, marijuana use, and other illicit drug use during pregnancy;[38] more likely to be pregnant in adolescence;[39] and more likely to report prenatal medical complications and infant complications post-delivery.[40]

Another study also demonstrated that ACE-surviving women were at increased risk for amenorrhea, which in this case was defined as missing one or more menstrual periods without being pregnant. They were also at increased risk for fertility difficulties, such as are seen in polycystic ovarian syndrome and other reproductive concerns. They were less likely to get pregnant in a single menstrual cycle and less likely to achieve a live birth in a single cycle. They had diminished ovarian reserve and function and an increased time to pregnancy (e.g. as a group, it took them longer to get pregnant than it took their non-ACE-surviving counterparts).[41] The associations between ACE score and reproductive health outcomes in this study remained significant, even when the researchers controlled for or leveled the playing field as it relates to age, body mass index, race, education, smoking, and income level.

Abuse And Reproductive Health Risks

The most frequently studied ACEs in connection with reproductive health are physical, sexual, and emotional abuse. Because researchers commonly study women who have suffered childhood abuse without asking about the other ACEs, we have a comparatively large body of research that looks at abuse in particular and how it affects reproductive health.

In one study conducted specifically on women who had experienced physical and/or sexual abuse, researchers demonstrated that those women who experienced physical abuse, sexual abuse, or both during childhood were more likely to have suicidal thoughts during pregnancy.[42] Additionally, women who experienced sexual abuse or both physical and sexual abuse were more likely to make at least one suicidal attempt prior to pregnancy.

In another study, researchers demonstrated that women who had experienced physical or emotional abuse were more likely to be obese prior to pregnancy.[43] Additional studies demonstrated increased risk of leiomyomas or fibroids in women who had experienced sexual or physical abuse,[44] and that women who had experienced childhood emotional, physical, or sexual abuse were at increased risk of experiencing pre-menstrual syndrome (PMS) symptoms,[45] which include symptoms like anxiety, mood swings, sadness, fatigue, bloating, breast tenderness, poor concentration, and food cravings.

CHAPTER 5 FEMALE PARTS

In a study that came out of Finland, women who had survived childhood abuse, including physical, sexual, and emotional abuse, were found to have a slightly increased risk of emergency Cesarean section (C-section) after the onset of labor (but not before), compared to women who did not experience abuse.[46] In considering the conclusion of this study, we need to keep in mind that the climates surrounding labor and delivery are very different in the United States and Finland. For example, when it comes to C-section rates, Finland has one of the lowest overall rates in Europe, with 16.2% of pregnant women delivering by C-section.[47] For comparison, the Center for Disease Control reports that 31.9% of deliveries in the United States are by C-section.[48] Given the fact that the C-section rate in the US is almost double that of Finland, I'd be interested in seeing whether and how the rate of C-section for women who have survived ACEs in the US differs from the rate of C-section for ACE-surviving Finnish women.

Here are a few of the available statistics from various studies:

- The children of women who reported one ACE had an average birth weight of 0.576 ounces lower than the children of women who reported no ACEs. Each additional ACE that the mothers experienced was associated with an additional 0.576-ounce decrease in the average birth weight of the children.[37]

- Women who experienced sexual and physical abuse in childhood and/or adolescence were more likely to be diagnosed with uterine fibroids in adulthood. Specifically, compared to women who did not experience abuse, women who experienced mild to moderate abuse of a single type (e.g. only physical or only sexual abuse) were 108% as likely, those who experienced mild abuse of multiple types or severe abuse of a single type were 117% as likely, those who experienced moderate abuse of a chronic nature or moderate abuse of multiple types were 123% as likely, those who experienced severe abuse of a chronic nature or multiple types of severe abuse were 124% as likely, and those who experienced multiple types of severe chronic abuse were 136% as likely as those who did not experience abuse to be diagnosed with fibroids in later life.[45]

- Women who reported the highest level of emotional abuse were 2.6 times as likely to experience PMS symptoms compared to those who did not report emotional abuse.[44]

- Women who reported severe physical abuse during childhood were 2.1 times as likely to report PMS symptoms, compared to those who did not report physical abuse.[44]

- Teen pregnancy occurred in 16%, 21%, 26%, 29%, 32%, 40%, 43%, and 53% of those with zero, one, two, three, four, five, six, and seven to eight ACEs, respectively.[39]

ACEs And Fertility

ACEs play an important role in fertility. Specifically, the changes that take place within the HPA axis in response to childhood trauma lead to suppression of some of our reproductive processes, including a decrease in many of the hormones that are essential for optimal reproductive health, such as estrogen and progesterone.

As women, we are not all equally fertile. Factors such as how regularly or consistently we ovulate, functionality of our fallopian tubes, whether and to what degree there is scar tissue or endometrial tissue present in our bodies, and other factors significantly impact fertility. In addition to varying from woman to woman, each of our fertility levels varies throughout our lifetime. For example, generally speaking, fertility begins to decline for women in our mid-thirties,[49] but age isn't the only factor that causes fertility to vary throughout our lifetimes.

Some of the research suggests that our degree of fertility also varies in a manner that reflects our stress levels. As an example, as the costs associated with raising children and the availability of resources change, our degree of fertility may reflect these changes. This is one of the reasons why it's possible for a woman to feel like it was so easy to get pregnant the first time, but then have a difficult time conceiving with subsequent attempts.

The fact that our fertility tends to reflect our stress levels (and more accurately, our HPA-axis function) is important to our understanding of ACE-related reproductive changes.

Allow me to explain. In a study that included over 9,000 women ages 18 and above at a primary care clinic in San Diego, California, researchers asked participants about the ACEs they had experienced and how old they were when they got pregnant the first time.[39] They also asked about some markers of stress levels, including whether or not each woman had experienced family problems, financial problems, job problems, uncontrollable anger, or felt like she was under high stress.

In order to analyze the data, they divided the women into four groups. The first group consisted of women with an ACE score of 0, the second consisted of women with an ACE score of 1 or 2, the third consisted of those with a score of 3 or 4, and the final group consisted of women with a score of 5 or greater. At the conclusion of the study, researchers found an association between each of these concerns and the participants' ACE scores. To be more specific, for every category of life stressors, the odds of experiencing that particular type of problem (e.g. family problems, financial problems, etc.) increased as the ACE score increased.

Furthermore, researchers found that, in and of itself and in the absence of ACEs, adolescent pregnancy did not increase the risk for these stressors. By comparing women who were pregnant during adolescence but experienced no ACEs to women who were pregnant during adolescence but did experience ACEs, researchers concluded that it was actually experiencing ACEs and not being pregnant during adolescence that was associated with an increased risk for life stressors.

ACEs, Feeling Stressed, And Reproductive Health

The fact that ACEs increase our risk for significant levels of perceived life stress is important because it is crucial to our understanding of the two ways that ACEs negatively impact our reproductive health.

First of all, we already know that ACEs lead to hyperactivity of the HPA axis, which is characterized by high levels of cortisol. The cortisol and other hormones involved in HPA-axis activation lead to alterations in our HPG axes and increase our risk for reproductive health concerns such as PMS, PCOS-like symptoms and other menstrual irregularities, and uterine fibroids. These HPG axis alterations can also affect our families and unborn children through increased risk for impaired fertility, prenatal medical complications, lower birth weight, and infant complications post-delivery.

Now, on top of this increased risk that we already carry for poor reproductive health because of the changes that took place with our HPA axes in early life, as female ACE survivors we are more likely than women who have not experienced ACEs (all other things being equal) to experience problems with our families, finances, jobs, managing our anger, and high stress levels. These types of problems can negatively affect our reproductive health as well. This is because when we experience life stressors, cortisol levels increase in order to help us face the stressors. As in the previous explanation, this increased activation of the stress response leads to HPG axis dysfunction, which leads to reproductive health concerns.

To summarize, childhood trauma leads to HPA-axis dysfunction and an increase in perceived life stress, both of which lead to elevations in cortisol and other stress hormones. These hormones exert an inhibitory effect on many of the HPG axis reproductive hormones, and this leads to reproductive health concerns in ACE-surviving women.

When we consider these facts together, we begin to see our dire need to address our increased risk in order to support optimal reproductive and overall health. When we discuss my B.A.L.A.N.C.E. Framework™, we'll talk about ways that you can mitigate your risk and start living your healthiest life now, for both yourself and your children.

CHAPTER 6

FRIENDLY FIRE

....

*How ACEs turn your immune system
into a loose canon that's turned on itself*

F atigue, hair loss, skin problems, anxiety, depression, joint pain and swelling, heart palpitations, swollen glands, digestive issues, abdominal pain, etc.—what do these widespread concerns have in common? And, even more importantly, what do they have to do with adverse childhood experiences?

The concerns I've listed are some of the most common symptoms of autoimmune disease. I strategically chose to start this chapter by listing some of the most prevalent symptoms of autoimmune disorders instead of listing some of the most common autoimmune diagnoses because many women reading this book will have experienced some of these symptoms, but they may not have ever been diagnosed with or even considered the possibility of having an autoimmune disease.

Survey data shows that, on average, women see five different doctors over the course of more than four years before they actually receive an accurate autoimmune diagnosis. What's even more interesting is the fact that many of the women who completed the survey stated that before they encountered a doctor who actually took the time to listen to their concerns and search for the source of those concerns, they were labeled as "chronic complainers."[50]

As ACE-surviving women, this information is important to us because our stressful childhood environments actually predispose us to autoimmune disease. The stress hormone cortisol is essential for immune system function in that after the immune system has been activated by a virus, bacterium, or something else, glucocorticoids like cortisol play a crucial role in turning off the immune response and bringing the body back to its normal state. If cortisol levels are elevated for prolonged periods of time, however, such as when we're exposed to chronic stress, including childhood trauma, it has a detrimental effect on the immune system.

We saw that when we experience ACEs, our HPA axes can be reprogrammed in such a way that they become hyperactive. When this occurs, cortisol levels rise, both at baseline when we're not particularly stressed and during acute and chronic stress. This eventually affects our inflammation levels and our immune systems as a whole.

ACEs And How Inflammation Levels Rise

When our HPA axes become hyperactive and cortisol levels rise, our inflammation levels begin to increase over time. This is because of the effect of prolonged cortisol exposure on what is referred to as the inflammatory reflex. To help you understand the inflammatory reflex, I'm going to use a somewhat simplified analogy. For the purposes of this analogy, I want you to think of the brain as a parent and inflammation as children. I also want you to think of the upper limit of normal inflammation levels, which is essentially the highest level that the brain will permit inflammation levels to rise to and still be considered normal, as a fence.

To keep them safe and healthy, parents allow their children to play either inside the house or outside in the backyard, but they have a fence up that protects them from venturing into unsafe territory. In the same way, there is a range of inflammation levels that is considered to be normal and the brain permits the body to have inflammation levels within that range without intervening.

Now, when cortisol levels are increased as a result of HPA-axis hyperactivation, what happens in the body is similar to what would happen if the fence were to be broken down or otherwise removed. Just as the children would be able to run more freely into unsafe areas, the restraint that the brain places on inflammation would be removed and the body's inflammation levels would increase to higher and potentially abnormal and unhealthy levels.

Just as the children would become accustomed to venturing farther and farther away from home without the fence, when the restraints placed on inflammation levels are removed by HPA-axis dysregulation, the body becomes accustomed to having higher and higher levels of inflammation. In other words, higher cortisol levels such as occurs as a result of ACE exposure remove the normal physiological restraints placed on the body by the inflammatory reflex,[51] and this leads to a tendency toward higher inflammation levels within the body.[52]

As a result of this physiological phenomenon, many ACE survivors develop elevated inflammatory markers (such as elevated C-reactive protein), and these abnormal values can persist for up to 20 years after we are removed from the stressful environment.[4] This predisposes us to conditions of immune system dysregulation such as auto-immune diseases.

Research suggests that this increased risk for auto-immune disease affects females more than males. As women, we are at increased risk for this process taking place because we naturally have higher levels of glucocorticoids (such as cortisol) at baseline than men do. One of the reasons for this phenomenon is estrogen's effect on the HPA-axis hormone CRH and on the immune system chemical messenger interleukin-4, also referred to as IL-4. IL-4 increases our risk for rheumatological autoimmune diseases like lupus, rheumatoid arthritis, scleroderma, and Sjögren's above other forms of auto-immune conditions. This may explain why conservative estimates suggest that up to 80% of people diagnosed with these types of autoimmune diseases are females.[4]

ACEs And Autoimmune Disease Risk

So far, we have research demonstrating a clear correlation between adverse childhood experiences and the following autoimmune diseases: autoimmune thrombocytopenia purpura, dermatomyositis, diabetes mellitus type 1, Grave's disease, Hashimoto's thyroiditis, idiopathic myocarditis, idiopathic pulmonary fibrosis, myesthenia gravis, rheumatoid arthritis, scleroderma, Sjögren's, systemic lupus erythematosus, ulcerative colitis, and Wegener's granulomatosis.[4]

Research also demonstrates a correlation between ACEs and both myalgic encephalomyelitis/chronic fatigue syndrome (ME/CFS) and fibromyalgia—two conditions that aren't autoimmune in nature but that have similar symptoms to many autoimmune disorders—with ACE survivors being two to three times more likely to be diagnosed with ME/CFS or fibromyalgia.

Here are a few of the available statistics from one large-scale study:[4]

- Researchers noted a significant relationship between ACE score and likelihood of a first hospitalization in women for any autoimmune disease. Specifically, women who had experienced two or more ACEs were significantly more likely to be hospitalized for any autoimmune disease compared to women who experienced one ACE or none. The relationship also existed for men, but it was not statistically significant.

- Compared with those with no ACEs, people with two or more ACEs were 70% more likely to be diagnosed with and hospitalized for T-helper 1- (Th1-) type autoimmune diseases, including type-1 diabetes, idiopathic myocarditis, idiopathic pulmonary fibrosis, ulcerative colitis, and Wegener's granulomatosis.

- Compared with those with no ACEs, people with two or more ACEs were 80% more likely to be diagnosed with and hospitalized for T-helper 2- (Th2-) type autoimmune diseases, including autoimmune thrombocytopenia purpura, Grave's disease, Hashimoto's thyroiditis, and Myesthenia gravis.

- Compared with those with no ACEs, people with two or more ACEs were 100% more likely to be diagnosed with and hospitalized for rheumatic autoimmune diseases, including dermatomyositis, rheumatoid arthritis, scleroderma, Sjögren's, and systemic lupus erythematosus.

- Analysis of the data revealed a 20% increased risk for Th1-type autoimmune disease, 20% increased risk for Th2-type autoimmune disease, and 30% increased risk for rheumatic diseases for each additional ACE level (e.g. 1 ACE, 2 ACEs, or 3+ ACEs) compared to 0 ACEs.

- Note: some autoimmune disorders, including Addison disease, autoimmune hemolytic anemia, Celiac disease, multiple sclerosis, pernicious anemia, psoriasis, and vitiligo elicit mixed Th1 and Th2 responses. In this particular study, researchers did not observe any clear association between ACEs and hospitalizations due to mixed Th1- and Th2-type autoimmune diseases.

What Does This Increased Risk Really Mean?

To effectively explain the statistics I've shared, it's important for us to discuss what being 100% more likely to be diagnosed with and hospitalized for a health condition does and does not mean. I want to make it clear that the 100% increased risk of being hospitalized with rheumatic autoimmune disease does *not* mean that a person will definitely be diagnosed with this type of autoimmune disease in their lifetime. There are several other factors at play here, such as epigenetics, hormones, smoking status, diet, environmental toxin exposure, social interactions, and the makeup of our gastrointestinal microbiome, and these factors can either lead to increased risk or help protect you from these autoimmune diseases.

Instead, a 100% increased risk in this case means that, as a group, people who have experienced two or more ACEs are 100% as likely, or to put it more simply, twice as likely to be hospitalized with rheumatic autoimmune diseases as people of similar demographics who have not experienced trauma.

This isn't exactly what it means since the calculated risk is based on averages of a group, and we're trying to convert that percentage to individual risk, but you wouldn't be too far off if you thought of it this way: If a woman's risk of being hospitalized with lupus, for example, had she not experienced abuse, given all of her physiological and lifestyle factors, was 4%, because she experienced this trauma, her risk is now increased by 100%, making it 8%.

In other words, if your ACE score is 2 or higher, the 100% increased risk you carry for rheumatic autoimmune diseases can be thought of as your risk being doubled as a result of the trauma you've experienced, not as you being unavoidably destined to be diagnosed with one.

How The Immune System Works

To help you further understand exactly how ACEs influence the immune system, I need to explain how the immune system functions normally. To do this, let's use a very simplistic analogy of the US Navy. In the Navy, the average soldier is trained for combat under a variety of different circumstances. When there's a very unique or specific mission, however, that calls for Special Forces—the specially trained Navy Seals are deployed to accomplish this mission. This is similar to how our immune systems function.

CHAPTER 6 FRIENDLY FIRE

The immune system can be divided into two branches: the non-specific or innate immune system and the specific or adaptive immune system. As the names suggest, we are born with our innate immune systems, but our adaptive immune systems—the special forces—are developed when we are exposed to new foreign invaders.

The innate immune system springs into action when we first come into contact with a foreign invader, regardless of whether that invader is a bacterium, virus, or some other pathogen. The special forces, on the other hand, are deployed under different circumstances. The adaptive immune system involves lymphocytes, a type of white blood cell, and these lymphocytes are divided into two classes: B cells and T cells. They come into play when the invader has been identified and the body is able to take a more precise approach to defeating the enemy.

Here's a note about the key players in the adaptive immune system: B cells play a crucial role in the process of engaging the body's special forces. Viruses, bacteria, and other pathogens have specific "antigens" on the outside that can bind to proteins. Think of these antigens as puzzle pieces that can bind to antibodies. Each B cell has antibodies on its outside that can bind to one specific antigen. For example, B cell X will not bind to the same antigen that B cell Z will. T cells, on the other hand, are like officers in the armed forces. They can direct and enhance the immune response, but they can also be engaged in combat under specific circumstances—in this case, when the body's own cells become infected or cancerous.

Let's see how this all plays out. When we're cut and come into contact with a specific germ for the first time, the innate immune system springs into action and the regular forces begin trying to destroy the invader. They don't stop to ask questions. What's the identity of this germ? Is it a bacterium? virus? parasite? They only know that it doesn't belong in the body and they non-specifically begin the process of blocking, deterring, or destroying the invader.

At the same time, thousands of B cells are "bumping" into the invader over the course of several days to see if its puzzle piece or antigen will bind to their particular antibodies. When a B cell bumps into the invader and its antibody binds to the invader's antigen, then something amazing happens. A T cell comes by to check if the B cell truly is bound to the antigen of the invader, and if it is, the B cell becomes activated.

The B cell becoming activated equates to the body finding out that we're dealing with a staph infection and not some other type of infection. Now that we know the nature of the enemy, the special forces—the specific or adaptive immune system—are ramped up. The B cell that has the antibodies that bind to the antigen of the current invader rapidly clones itself, making two types of cells: plasma cells, which are B cells that will then produce more antibodies to that specific antigen and release them into the circulation so that they can bind to the invaders and mark them for destruction, and memory cells, which remember the pattern of the invader's antigen so that the adaptive immune system can come into effect faster and destroy the enemy sooner in the event that the pathogen invades again in the future. As a part of our adaptive immunity, if our own cells become infected by foreign invaders or cancerous, T cells can also play an important role in destroying those cells that are no longer serving the body.

Chronic Stress And Autoimmune Disease

Now that we have a more complete understanding of how the immune system functions, I'll summarize how chronic childhood stress affects the immune system and explain how both our childhood and adulthood stress levels affect our autoimmune risk.

When we first come into contact with a stressor, the acute stress up-regulates portions of the innate immune system, leading to increased inflammation. Cortisol and other glucocorticoids then work to quiet the hyperactive immune system. If the stressor persists, the adrenal glands continue to secrete cortisol, and this leads to the suppression of various aspects of both the innate and adaptive portions of the immune system.

Elevated cortisol levels lead to problems with cortisol signaling, which is essentially where cortisol has a harder time feeding back to the brain and other cells and turning off the stress and immune responses. Elevated cortisol levels also remove the normal physiological restraints placed on the body by the vagus nerve's inflammatory reflex, and this leads to a tendency toward higher inflammation levels within the body. The result is elevated inflammatory markers that can continue for up to 20 years after you are removed from the stressful environment and predisposes you for conditions of immune system dysregulation, such as autoimmune diseases.

This process of stress-induced immune system-related changes predisposing us to autoimmune diseases is relevant to both childhood and adulthood stress. This is because when we experience stress in adulthood, it actually suppresses our immune systems in a similar manner to how ACEs affect our immune systems. While stress in adulthood is less likely to actually change our HPA axes, it can lead to elevations in cortisol levels and increase our risk of being diagnosed with an autoimmune disease as a result. In fact, up to 80% of adults who were diagnosed with one or more autoimmune diseases reported an abnormally high level of emotional and psychological stress immediately prior to being diagnosed.[53] This is why stress is such an important risk factor for autoimmune diseases.

Now that you understand how ACEs affect your risk for autoimmune disease, I want you to take courage. When we talk about my B.A.L.A.N.C.E. Framework™, we'll discuss ways to decrease stress levels and how I address many of the other risk factors for autoimmune diseases that I've mentioned, such as epigenetics, hormones, diet, the gastrointestinal microbiome, and more.

CHAPTER 7

WESTERN KILLERS

....

How fast food and sedentary lifestyles might not be the full story on the common killer diseases

When our innate immune systems are activated in response to childhood and other types of psychological stressors, the activation process is very similar to what takes place when a virus or bacterium is invading the body. Yet this inflammatory process is not localized to our immune systems. Instead, as part of the stress response, epinephrine, cortisol, and other stress hormones induce an inflammatory process known as an acute phase response, and this inflammatory process actually causes structural changes in our cardiovascular systems, specifically in our arteries.[54]

This inflammatory process is the foundation of a cluster of related concerns. These concerns include high triglyceride levels, low HDL cholesterol levels, increased blood pressure, high blood sugar, and excess body fat around the waist. If a person has three or more of these concerns, we say they have metabolic syndrome, or syndrome X.

Because of the inflammatory processes that take place in our bodies as ACE survivors, we are at increased risk for metabolic syndrome. Metabolic syndrome increases our risk for cardiovascular disease, diabetes, and death from these and other causes, but the good news is that metabolic syndrome is preventable and, in the vast majority of cases, completely reversible.

ACEs And Cardiovascular Disease

There are two reasons why this is important to us as ACE survivors. The first is that most people begin to develop atherosclerosis or plaque in their arteries by their teens and twenties.[55] This plaque buildup begins before we can see changes in the high cholesterol blood tests your doctor does each year, so it's not uncommon to have a buildup of atherosclerotic plaque and yet have perfect blood cholesterol levels.

The second reason this is important to us as ACE survivors is related to the fact that, because of the inflammatory process it induces, psychological stress damages the integrity of our arteries. Here are the details: If you've already begun to develop plaque buildup in your arteries, which again begins in the teens or twenties for most people, and then you are exposed to a chronic psychological stressor, then the inflammatory and structural changes to your artery walls that come about as a result of activation of the stress response become even more exaggerated and can lead to further damage to the blood vessels.

This inflammatory process and the compounded effect that comes about when we experience ACEs after atherosclerosis has already begun to set in explain how childhood trauma, in combination with increased stress levels in youth and adulthood, increases ACE survivors' risk for developing cardiovascular disease. This includes heart attack, stroke, heart failure, coronary artery disease, peripheral artery disease, and other forms of atherosclerosis and cardiovascular disease, and the association between ACEs and these cardiovascular concerns persists, even when we control for the factors that typically increase cardiovascular risk.[56]

ACEs And Blood Pressure

Unfortunately, this isn't the end of the story. Imagine you have a specific garden hose that you typically use. It's your favorite one to use because the water pressure comes out just right. Now imagine you try to turn on your water to use the hose, but you notice a difference in pressure—perhaps the water only trickles or doesn't come out at all. You turn the water off to investigate, only to find that your curious toddler has placed a rock or some dirt into the hose. Because of this obstruction, the pressure inside of the hose began to build up when you turned on the water.

Now, what does this have to do with our discussion on metabolic syndrome and adverse childhood experiences? Well, this hose analogy is very similar to how atherosclerosis affects your blood pressure. When plaque accumulates in your arteries, whether it is through high stress levels, poor dietary choices, or some other cause, the plaque decreases the available space in your arteries, much like the rock or dirt did with the hose.

This narrowing of the arteries leads to an increase in the pressure of the blood that is being pumped from your heart to the rest of your body. Therefore, ACEs not only increase your risk for atherosclerosis, but they also increase your risk for hypertension or high blood pressure, and we can see this increase in blood pressure as early as young adulthood.[57]

Increases in blood pressure also increase the degree of inflammation in the walls of the arteries,[54] which leads to increased atherosclerosis, and the cycle continues.

ACEs And Blood Sugar

Our bodies convert glucose into energy. Whether we are being prepared to fight or flee oncoming danger, we need energy to accomplish our goals. In order to meet this need, when our stress hormones like cortisol rise, they increase the amount of glucose that is present in our bloodstreams. Essentially, our stress hormones increase our blood sugar so that we can use that sugar to produce energy in order to face the stressor at hand.

Insulin, a hormone that is produced by the beta cells of the pancreas, has the opposite effect. While stress hormones like epinephrine and cortisol increase blood sugar, insulin lowers blood sugar by enabling the glucose to be stored in our muscles, fat cells, and liver for later use or by converting it to energy. You may have heard narratives that have painted insulin in a bad light, but I want you to understand that insulin is not the bad guy here; our bodies need insulin to function properly.

Because insulin and stress hormones like cortisol have opposing effects, it is well known that prolonged stress frequently results in the development of insulin resistance.[54] Insulin resistance is essentially a state in which insulin is still present within the body but, for one reason or another, the body does not respond to it in the way that it should. Because the body becomes resistant to insulin, it requires higher and higher levels of insulin to send the glucose into the cells and keep the amount of sugar that is present in the bloodstream within the normal range.

Insulin resistance is problematic because our bodies always want to be in a state of balance. As the insulin resistance progresses, it becomes more and more difficult for the body to compensate for the increasing blood sugar levels; the body has a harder time keeping blood sugar levels within the normal range. This frequently results in glucose intolerance (also referred to as hyperglycemia or pre-diabetes) and then it progresses to diabetes mellitus type 2.

Uncontrolled type-2 diabetes can come along with a host of unwanted complications, including kidney damage, vision loss, nerve damage, poor wound healing, and depression. It also significantly increases our risk for cognitive decline and Alzheimer's disease.

Insulin's Role In The HPA Axis

In addition to controlling blood sugar, insulin plays a significant role in activating the stress response. This is because it has important effects on the HPA axis.[9]

You already know that when we are exposed to ACEs, our HPA axes tend to initially become hyperactive, and our bodies have exaggerated responses to stress as a result. If this continues for an extended period of time, the body begins to have a decreased response to stress hormones, and the HPA axis becomes hypoactive. It's like we're numb at this point; it becomes more difficult for our bodies to mount a stress response. This is typically seen in people with post-traumatic stress disorder, which affects 5–10% of the United States population.[58]

This is relevant to our current discussion because insulin helps regulate the HPA axis. When our bodies become resistant to insulin, the HPA axis responds less to insulin and the stress response becomes abnormal. In other words, insulin resistance leads to dysregulation of the HPA axis in both ACE survivors and our non-ACE-surviving counterparts. In the case of ACE survivors, the HPA axis becomes even more abnormal than it was previously because we already have to deal with the trauma-induced changes that occurred with our HPA axes during childhood.

This link between metabolic concerns like diabetes and HPA-axis dysregulation is important because it shows how, as ACE survivors, our risk for chronic physical and mental health concerns compounds. Because this process leads to further HPA-axis dysregulation, it increases our risk for depression and other mental health concerns, and this explains why diabetic individuals and those with varying degrees of insulin resistance are at increased risk for depression, compared to individuals with optimal blood sugar control.[9]

ACEs And Weight Control

The relationship between adverse childhood experiences and weight is somewhat complex. On one hand, catecholamines like epinephrine increase the breakdown of fatty deposits within the body, leading to fat loss.[54] Because epinephrine release is an important part of our acute stress response activation process, this partly explains why some people lose weight when they are under lots of stress.

Let's look at the subject from another angle to help us visualize how complex the relationship between weight and childhood trauma is. You already know that our HPA axes can become hyperactivated in response to ACE exposure and that, after some time of continuing under these circumstances, the body sometimes attempts to compensate for the increase in stress hormones by decreasing the available amount of our stress hormone receptors. Remember my analogy with the hormones as keys and receptors as locks? This is another place where it comes into play. The stress hormones, which we're thinking of as keys, have been activating the stress response or unlocking the doors so frequently that the body attempts to compensate for this hyperactivation by removing some of the locks from the doors, which in this case is a representation of the CRH hormone receptors at the level of the pituitary gland.

This downregulation of our stress hormone receptors, or removal of the locks in an attempt to prevent the hyperactivation that was taking place, results in a secondary hypoactivation of the HPA axis. Now, instead of overreacting to everything that the body perceives as stressful, our bodies find it difficult to mount a normal stress response, even when we are exposed to serious stressors.

Under these circumstances, the effect of our ACEs on our weight tend to take a different form. When our HPA axes become hypoactive, such as occurs when our hormone receptors are downregulated after prolonged exposure to stress hormones, we begin to accumulate fat. This is because our bodies are now comparatively deprived of the stimulation of these fat-reducing stress hormones.

To further complicate the relationship between ACEs and weight, high stress levels are likely a major factor in overeating. In other words, for many people, eating when stressed provides a welcome distraction from psychological stressors and provides a sensation of temporary relief.

Furthermore, we know that elevated cortisol levels lead to an increase in abdominal fat, so when we are under chronic stress for a prolonged period of time, our belly fat tends to increase.

With these and other factors coming in to play, the way that our ACEs affect our weight tends to vary from one person to another. Let's look at some of the research and see what conclusions we can draw.

ACEs And Weight Research

One study found that men who experienced ACEs in childhood were more likely to be overweight or obese in adulthood, and while it didn't note this correlation in women, the study found that women who experienced ACEs were more likely to skip meals to lose weight or have other problematic eating habits.[59] Another study noted an increased likelihood of being obese, being underweight, or exhibiting extreme weight loss behaviors in ACE-surviving girls relative to their non-ACE-surviving counterparts.

The type of ACEs they experienced seemed to impact their risk. Those who had experienced sexual abuse were more likely to be obese and to demonstrate extreme weight loss behaviors. Those who had experienced physical lack, such as in the case of parental unemployment, were more likely to be either obese or underweight. And those who witnessed an unwinding of the family fabric, such as in the case of witnessing domestic violence or losing a parent, were more prone to excessive exercise or other extreme weight loss behaviors.[60] Furthermore, another study found that women who experienced physical or emotional abuse were more likely to be overweight prior to becoming pregnant, relative to non-ACE-surviving women.[43]

This wide array of predispositions in females, with the correlations being contingent upon the nature of the ACEs experienced, provides us with a potential explanation of why the previous study, which grouped all ACEs together and looked for a correlation between them and obesity, was not able to find one. It's likely that the increased risk of being underweight in some ACE survivors served to offset the increased risk of being overweight in others, making it difficult to draw a definitive conclusion that could be applied to all ACE-surviving women.

ACEs And Metabolic Disorder Risk

So far, the research demonstrates a clear correlation between adverse childhood experiences and the following metabolic concerns: hypertension,[61] heart attack, stroke, heart failure, coronary artery disease, peripheral artery disease, other forms of atherosclerosis and cardiovascular disease,[56] insulin resistance, pre-diabetes, type-2 diabetes mellitus,[54,58] disordered eating habits,[59] and being underweight, overweight, or obese.[59–60]

Here are a few of the available statistics from various studies:

- One study found that those who experienced four or more adverse childhood experiences had a twofold increased risk of severe obesity, defined as a Body Mass Index ≥ 35.[62]

- People who experienced ACEs were more likely to be diagnosed with type-2 diabetes, and every additional ACE was associated with an approximately 11% increase in odds of developing diabetes.[63]

- Compared to those who were raised in more favorable family environments, individuals who were exposed to less favorable family environments (e.g. experiences of abuse or neglect) were 129% to 153% more likely to experience a cardiovascular event, including fatal and non-fatal heart attack, stroke, heart failure, coronary artery disease, peripheral artery disease, and other fatal atherosclerotic or cardiovascular disease events.[56]

ACEs and How Psychiatric Medications Increase Risk

As ACE survivors, the underlying inflammatory process that is taking place in our bodies predisposes us to metabolic syndrome, but this isn't our only source of increased risk. Our increased risk for metabolic syndrome is compounded by the fact that those of us with an ACE score of 5 or more are three times more likely to be prescribed antidepressants and ten times more likely to be prescribed antipsychotics, compared to those who have not experienced ACEs.[29]

The reason why this statistic is relevant is that the United States Food and Drug Administration currently requires that all atypical antipsychotics, including Zyprexa (olanzapine), Clozaril (clozapine), Seroquel (quetiapine), Abilify (aripiprazole), Risperdal (risperidone), and others carry a warning that they increase the risk for hyperglycemia and diabetes. This is because, although some increase our risk more than others do,[64] all of the antipsychotic drugs that are currently available increase our risk for high blood sugar to some degree.

Additionally, antidepressant medication, such as serotonin-specific reuptake inhibitors (SSRIs) and serotonin-norepinephrine reuptake inhibitors (SNRIs), may also increase the risk for metabolic syndrome,[33] which we saw includes high triglyceride levels, low HDL cholesterol levels, increased blood pressure, high blood sugar, and excess body fat around the waist.

When we discuss my B.A.L.A.N.C.E. Framework™, we'll learn things we can do to curb our increased risk so we can live our healthiest and best lives now, in spite of our past.

CHAPTER 8

FIND B.A.L.A.N.C.E.

....

The ultimate guide to effective, comprehensive ACE treatment to help get on the road to recovery fast

Now that we've discussed the four major categories of health conditions for which we are at increased risk as ACE survivors and the science of how this increased risk comes about, it's time for some hope. In this chapter, I'll share my B.A.L.A.N.C.E. Framework™ and how we, as female ACE survivors, can use it to preserve or regain our health so that we can live life on our own terms, raise physically and emotionally resilient children, rise above our past and present circumstances, and live our healthiest and best lives now, in spite of our past experiences.

Before we delve into the framework, I want to make sure you understand a very crucial point: Just as these categories of concerns have a common psychological cause, in this case ACEs, they also have a common biological or physiological cause, which in this case is the physical effects that ACEs have on the body, namely HPA-axis dysregulation, structural changes that take place within the brain, and increased inflammation.

Throughout my years of medical school and helping patients in my own private practice, I have learned by experience that the most lasting way to address a health concern and get the most consistent and desirable results in the long run is to address the underlying cause of the concern at the same time that we are providing symptomatic relief by helping to address the most pressing symptoms.

Here's an example of what I mean: I have an uncle who is a real estate investor and renovator and I've seen him do this type of work, so I like to think of it this way. If the foundation of your house begins to settle or shift, and if the walls begin to crack and the house is affected as a result, you could hire someone to come in and modify the walls by filling in the cracks and then repainting them.

That would definitely work for some time, but as the foundation continued to shift and new cracks appeared in the walls, you'd need to continually modify them by filling in the new cracks and repainting, possibly for the rest of your lifetime in that house. But how much better would it be if instead of addressing the foundational shifts as you see them manifested as cracks in the walls of the house, you do what my uncle does and address the problem at the house's foundation? Of course, it would be a lot more work in the beginning, but wouldn't the results be far better in the long run? Wouldn't you be happier in the long run?

Addressing ACE-related health concerns is very similar to this house scenario. If, as an ACE survivor, you're diagnosed with diabetes, we could put you on metformin to get your blood sugar down. We could. However, if it doesn't normalize your sugar as much as we had hoped it would, we'll end up increasing the dosage or adding additional medication as modifications, further increasing your risk for side effects that will also need to be addressed.

If you later become depressed, a common complication of diabetes, and we attempt to support your mood by giving you an SSRI like Lexapro (escitalopram), then we may address your mood, but we'll also likely further increase your risk for metabolic syndrome.[65] As the syndrome progresses, we may even end up adding another modification in the form of Lipitor (atorvastatin) or some other medication to lower your now-elevated cholesterol, all without ever addressing the problem at its core.

If, however, instead of going the route of adding modifications, we decide to address your concern at its foundation, it may require more work in the beginning, but we'd significantly reduce the amount of problems that may arise in the future.

Think of the four major categories of ACE-related chronic disease—mental health concerns, reproductive concerns, autoimmune disorders, and metabolic concerns—as the four exterior walls of a house; they have a common foundation. When you understand this fact, you'll be better able to understand why the treatments for these four seemingly different categories of health concerns are so similar.

As ACE survivors, we can (and should) support optimal health at the foundational level by addressing HPA-axis dysregulation, brain changes, and inflammation and by addressing the damage that has already been done using minimally invasive modifications. Please note that addressing the damage that has already occurred at the time that we begin to address the foundation is fundamentally different from neglecting the foundation altogether and addressing future damage as it occurs.

When we simultaneously work at improving the foundation and correcting the damage that occurred in the past, we can effectively reduce our risk for these four categories of ACE-related health concerns and, in many cases, we can address and even reverse these conditions. I've seen this in my own practice.

This is where my B.A.L.A.N.C.E. Framework™ comes in. The B.A.L.A.N.C.E. Framework™ embodies the foundational work we need to do as ACE survivors to preserve and restore optimal health, as well as describes minimally invasive modifications that we can employ to address these four categories of health concerns while working on their foundation, whether they've recently begun to settle in or whether we've been dealing with them for several years.

I say it's hard work because it encompasses lifestyle modifications that address the core changes that take place within our brains and bodies and that are common to all affected ACE survivors, regardless of whether our symptoms manifest as mental health concerns, reproductive concerns, autoimmune disorders, metabolic concerns, or some combination of these concerns. Despite being hard work, though, I can tell you and my patients can attest to the fact that the results make it all worth it.

The B.A.L.A.N.C.E. Framework™

What exactly is the B.A.L.A.N.C.E. Framework™? B.A.L.A.N.C.E. is an acronym that stands for:

- Biomarker optimization
- Address genetic risk
- Lifestyle adjustments
- Address past trauma
- Normalize and/or optimize hormones
- Correct gut flora abnormalities
- Eliminate or reduce medication

I've used this framework to construct specific protocols and treatment plans for patients diagnosed with each of the four categories of health concerns for which we're at increased risk as ACE survivors. For example, my P7 Protocol™, which is the protocol I describe in detail in my book *Optimize Your Body, Heal Your Mind* and use to help patients overcome their mental health concerns, is based on this framework.

While there is some variation in the way I address each of these four types of concerns, I'm able to use my B.A.L.A.N.C.E. Framework™ over and over again to help ACE survivors support optimal health and address and reverse disease because the foundational physiological changes that predispose us to these concerns are the same across all four major categories of ACE-related chronic health conditions.

Because we've been talking about all four categories of ACE-related chronic disease, I'll share a brief overview of the B.A.L.A.N.C.E. Framework™, keeping things specific to the foundational information that is relevant to all four categories of diseases. I'll also place more emphasis on lifestyle-related therapeutics rather than herbs and supplements, because drug-herb and drug-nutrient interactions can be very serious, and it would be irresponsible for any healthcare professional to make specific recommendations that may end up being harmful to you because of the medication you are taking or the other conditions with which you've been diagnosed.

As always, I recommend working with a qualified healthcare professional who takes a functional and individualized approach to wellness and can monitor your progress in order to help address your diagnosed health concerns in a safe, holistic manner. Doing so helps to ensure that your wellness journey is as painless and smooth as possible.

Now that I've explained that, I'll share a brief overview of each of the seven aspects of this framework.

Biomarker Optimization

The term "biomarker" is actually a combination of the two words "biological" and "marker," and it simply means a measurable substance in an organism whose presence indicates some phenomenon such as disease, infection, or environmental exposure. Essentially, a biomarker is a substance that we can measure in blood, urine, saliva, stool, or some other sample type, and its presence, or in many cases, the degree to which it is present, tells us something about the state of the organism in which it is found. In this case, the biomarkers we'll be discussing provide us with objective information about our risk for disease as well as provide us with direction on how we can optimize our health.

The Importance of Biomarker Optimization-
One of the reasons why it's important for us to take a critical look at these wellness biomarkers is the fact that, in many cases, there is a crucial difference between the "normal" range and the "optimal" range. I'll use thyroid function as an example to explain what I mean.

We'll revisit the thyroid when we talk about normalizing and optimizing hormonal function, but here is what you need to know for the purposes of this illustration: The thyroid is a butterfly-shaped gland located in the front of the neck that controls growth and metabolism, among other things. In conventional medicine, thyroid function is usually checked by a blood test called thyroid-stimulating hormone, or TSH. The normal range for TSH varies slightly from lab to lab, but generally speaking, it is about 0.450 to 4.500 uIU/mL.

What's interesting about TSH is that the data from some pretty important studies[66] suggest that the "normal" or reference range for TSH isn't as reliable as we once thought. The authors of a National Health and Nutrition Examination Survey III-based study looked at the relationships between TSH and two types of thyroid antibodies in pregnant women. At the end of this study, researchers concluded that when we initially looked at thyroid function and came up with the "normal" values for the TSH reference range, we may have been wrong about the upper limit because some of the people who appeared to have healthy, well-functioning thyroid glands (and on whose lab values we based the normal range) may have actually been in the early stages of thyroid disease.

Thyroid function is relevant to mental and reproductive health, autoimmunity, and metabolic concerns. Here's just one clinical example of how poor thyroid health can affect us in one of these areas: We know that abnormal thyroid function can lead to recurrent miscarriages and other reproductive difficulties. Researchers wanted to find out if having a TSH value that was on the higher side of the reference range but still considered "normal" led to a difference in outcome for fertility treatments, compared to having an optimal TSH value.

They found that women who had TSH values above 2.5 uIU/mL got pregnant at a rate of 21.6%, while women with TSH values at 2.49 uIU/mL and below conceived at a rate of 56.6%—more than double that of their counterparts on the higher end of normal.[67] Keep in mind that the normal value for TSH is typically 0.45 to 4.50 uIU/mL (plus or minus 0.05). This indicates that, according to this "normal" range, women with a TSH of 2.5 uIU/mL are basically in the average or midline bracket. Yet these women with "average" thyroid function were suffering repercussions when it came to fertility, and this randomized, controlled clinical trial demonstrated that these difficulties correlated strongly with their suboptimal but apparently "normal" thyroid function.

To summarize, if you're trying to determine if your thyroid is functioning well and you turn to the "normal" range for guidance, you may actually be comparing your TSH value to a faulty standard. It would be sort of like trying to measure the weight of something using a scale that hasn't been calibrated or is a little off; it's not the best means of gathering the information you are seeking. This is why it's possible to have a TSH value that is technically within the normal range and still experience symptoms of suboptimal thyroid function.

Although I just used TSH as an example to explain the importance of looking at optimal ranges and not just the conventional reference ranges, this applies to many of our biomarkers as well. If we don't look at and aim for optimal values when it comes to our wellness biomarkers, we can end up with suboptimal health, not feeling our best and unsure why. This is why I advocate for ACE survivors using optimal ranges to evaluate important biomarkers of wellness; it sets the stage and builds a foundation for not just good, but optimal health.

When working with ACE survivors, I typically check and make recommendations to optimize biomarkers that are related to inflammation and therefore provide us with information about their risk for all four of the major categories of ACE-related chronic disease. These biomarkers include high-sensitivity C-reactive protein, homocysteine, omega 3 and 6 fatty acid profiles, and more. Because adverse childhood experiences lead to abnormalities with immune system function, including, as I shared with my fence analogy, a disinhibition or relaxing of the inflammatory reflex, higher levels of inflammation are very common in ACE survivors.

CHAPTER 8 FIND B.A.L.A.N.C.E.

These higher levels of inflammation wreak havoc on our health and, as we saw, are important physiological causative and/or contributing factors in mental health concerns, reproductive disorders, autoimmune diseases, and metabolic concerns. As a result, when we get a clear understanding of the role that inflammation plays in the development of various ACE-related chronic disease, it makes sense that looking at markers of inflammation and addressing abnormal or suboptimal values results in decreased risk for developing these conditions and overall improvements in many of these concerns.

Additionally, I look at biomarkers that provide us with information about general health, including glucose metabolism and kidney and liver function. This includes tests such as the complete blood count, comprehensive metabolic panel, vitamin D, the lipid (cholesterol) profile, hemoglobin a1c, and other tests that are relevant to us as ACE survivors. I also look at a few other lab tests, if indicated, such as an iron panel if they have symptoms of or their complete blood count suggests anemia, and labs that look at autoimmunity if they have symptoms of or have been diagnosed with autoimmune disease.

By checking each of these biomarkers with my patients and making recommendations to get them into the optimal range toward the beginning of our time together, I see substantial improvements in the way my patients feel, including accelerated improvements in mood, pain, and energy levels. I've found that assessing and addressing these biomarkers as early as possible through diet, lifestyle, and other minimally invasive therapies really allows us to create big shifts in the way the women with whom I work feel from the beginning of our time together.

Address Genetic Risk

As a part of the B.A.L.A.N.C.E. Framework™, I also assess genetic risk with ACE survivors. We look at genes that affect our abilities to handle and bounce back from stressful situations, genes that affect inflammation levels, genes that affect a process called methylation that impacts all four of the major categories of ACE-related chronic disease, genes that affect how our bodies process medication, and other relevant genes.

Just like experiencing negative stress during childhood can increase our risk for things like elevated inflammatory markers and decreased stress resilience, the genes that we inherit from our parents can further increase our risk,

CHAPTER 8 FIND B.A.L.A.N.C.E.

given the right (or wrong) environment. Our genes can also impact how we process different medications and whether and to what degree these medications will be effective in addressing our health concern.

By taking an in-depth look at ACE survivors' genetics, we're able to gain a deeper understanding of exactly why some of our biomarkers were outside the normal range and why you may not have gotten the response you desired when you started taking prescription medication. Most importantly, looking at your genetic makeup can provide us with valuable insight and further direction regarding where we need to focus our efforts in order to decrease your accumulated health risk.

I'll share just one example of how genetics can further increase our chronic disease risk as ACE survivors. Genes provide us with the instructions necessary to produce proteins and related molecules within the body. To understand what I'll be explaining, I want you to think of genes as colors in a 64-count crayon box. In this case, the red crayons represent one gene while the blue crayons represent another. Among the blue crayons, there is some variation. For example, there are royal blue, light blue, and even navy blue crayons. All these blue crayons represent one gene, which is completely separate from the gene represented by the red crayons, but the various shades within the blue category represent variations that exist within that particular gene from person to person.

Let's apply this analogy to an actual gene that exists within the human body. The FK506-binding protein 5 (FKBP5) gene provides your body with the instructions necessary to create a chaperone protein that controls the function of the receptors to which cortisol and similar hormones bind. Specifically, it modulates glucocorticoid receptor activity in response to stressors, helps regulate cortisol and glucocorticoid receptor sensitivity, and plays an important role in the termination of the stress response. Some people have variants of this gene that differ slightly in a specific spot from the default or most common version found within the population. We call these variations in the genes single nucleotide polymorphisms, or SNPs (pronounced "snips").

We can think of individuals who have these SNPs as having variations in the shade that is viewed as the norm when it comes to this gene. We're still talking about the FKBP5 gene, so this isn't a mutation in the gene that results in a non-functioning protein or a completely

CHAPTER 8 FIND B.A.L.A.N.C.E.

different protein altogether. In other words, the difference isn't great enough to be represented by a red crayon; instead, we're talking about a very minute difference that, although small, under certain circumstances (such as in the context of childhood trauma), can lead to epigenetic changes that can have big effects.

When it comes to the FKBP5 gene, I usually look at the rs1360780 SNP because it is one that has been shown to be very strongly associated with stress resilience, and also because ACE survivors who have the navy and light blue versions of this gene, and not the royal blue or common version, tend to have even greater risk for mental health, reproductive, autoimmune, and metabolic concerns, compared to the already increased risk that ACE survivors who have the coveted royal blue variant of this gene have.

Scientifically speaking, individuals with the CC version of this SNP have the default or "normal" version—think of it as being royal blue. On the other hand, those with the CT or TT version—think navy blue or light blue, respectively—have variants that are associated with less desirable outcomes. In fact, when compared with those who have the royal blue version of the gene, those who had the navy or light blue variants were more likely to have cortisol levels that did not return to the normal range after exposure to a stressor and reported higher levels of anxiety after being exposed to psychosocial stressors.[68] This translates to increased risk for elevated cortisol levels, decreased likelihood of managing stress in a healthy manner, and increased risk for all four categories of ACE-related chronic disease.

In cases where the ACE survivors with whom I work have FKBP5 variants that have been associated with insufficient cortisol recovery, I've found that they need additional emphasis on normalizing HPA-axis function and optimizing cortisol levels. To address this, I ensure that their vitamin D levels are at the higher end of the optimal range because research suggests that vitamin D may have a direct effect on FKBP5 expression.[69] I also use additional means such as phosphatidylserine and adaptogenic herbs like Ashwagandha to help optimize cortisol levels and support a healthy stress response, when indicated.[12, 70–71]

This illustration from the FKBP5 gene is just one example of how genetics can affect our risk for ACE-related chronic disease. As ACE survivors, genetics are important, but what is even more important is the epigenetic expression of our genes, which is essentially our genes being expressed more or less based on our interactions with our environments. The "environment" that influences our gene expression includes a variety of factors, such as social interactions, hormones, smoking history, diet, and environmental toxin exposure, as we'll see throughout my explanation of the B.A.L.A.N.C.E. Framework™.

As ACE survivors, the epigenetic expression of our genes can work either for or against us in our quests to obtain optimal health, and the first step toward supporting optimal wellness in cases where we have genes that increase our risk and allowing our beneficial genes to work for us is understanding our genes and the risks or benefits that they confer.

Lifestyle Adjustments

Lifestyle adjustments are a huge part of the B.A.L.A.N.C.E. Framework™. As much as people hate to hear it, the fact is that whether or not a person makes and faithfully adheres to appropriate lifestyle adjustments can really be a determining factor in whether they obtain optimal health for their age and circumstances in their lifetime.

When I address lifestyle with ACE survivors, I typically discuss five areas. I use the acronym N.E.E.D.S. to help my patients remember these five core areas—nature, exercise, environmental factors, diet, and sleep.

Nature-

One of the first lifestyle recommendations I make for ACE survivors is recommending that they spend time outdoors in nature. I make this lifestyle recommendation first because it is fairly easy to incorporate and it's associated with such positive results. Research demonstrates that being exposed to nature results in as much as an additional 21.3% drop per hour in salivary cortisol levels beyond any drop associated with cortisol's normal daily pattern.[72] Another study demonstrated that being exposed to natural environments led to a decrease in interleukin-6 and tumor necrosis factor alpha, two chemicals that are associated with a heightened inflammatory response in the body.[73]

Even more interesting is the fact that regardless of whether or not you are actually active while outdoors, spending time in natural environments can result in a decrease in cortisol and inflammation levels. Exposure to natural environments can lead to both decreased activation of the sympathetic nervous system[74] and improvements in HPA-axis function,[72] both of which result in decreased risk for ACE-related chronic disease.

If that sounds simple enough, it gets even better! The greatest decrease in cortisol levels per time spent outdoors was seen between the 20- and 30-minute marks. After 30 minutes, cortisol levels continued to decline with exposure to natural environments, but at a slower rate.

This means that even if you have just 20 to 30 minutes to spare, you can receive immense benefit, as far as reducing your risk for chronic disease is concerned, by spending that time, for example, outside sitting in your backyard instead of at a desk or on your bed inside.

Exercise-

When I shared the study on children in Romania who had suffered neglect as a result of their early environment, I mentioned that experiencing ACEs has been shown to lead to changes within the brain. These brain changes, specifically a decrease in brain volume, are characterized by a decrease in both gray and white matter. As a reminder, larger volumes of gray matter are associated with an increase in various skills and abilities, while more white matter is associated with faster information processing, so all things being equal, decreases in both gray and white matter would be associated with fewer advanced skills and abilities and decreased ability to quickly process information.

When I work with ACE survivors, I place special emphasis on exercise as a lifestyle adjustment, and this is because exercise, specifically aerobic exercise, has been shown to increase both gray and white matter in randomized controlled trials.[75] Interestingly, stretching and other non-aerobic exercises did not have this effect. This isn't to say that anaerobic exercises such as high-intensity interval training are useless; they definitely have their place, and I do recommend them when indicated, but they have not been shown to have the same effects on the brain that aerobic exercises such as brisk walking, cycling, and swimming have.

Furthermore, research demonstrates that aerobic exercise increases neurogenesis (the growth of new nervous tissue, including brain cells) within the hippocampus,[76] an area of the brain that has been demonstrated to be smaller than normal in some ACE-affected children[14] and that plays a major role in learning and memory. We believe that exercise is able to have this effect because it increases brain-derived neurotrophic factor, also known as BDNF, a protein that plays a significant role in the survival, growth, maturation, and maintenance of brain and other nerve cells.

Neuroplasticity is the brain's ability to reorganize itself by forming new neural connections. Because exercise stimulates neuroplasticity by promoting the expression of BDNF, it increases our brain's volume, enhances its ability to form new connections, and supports our ability to develop new thoughts and learn new behaviors. These are all very important for us as ACE-surviving women because they help counteract the negative effects of early childhood trauma on the brain. I typically recommend that the ACE survivors with whom I work engage in moderate-intensity aerobic exercise at least three times per week in order to harness the brain benefits associated with physical activity.

Environmental Factors-
Our physical environment has important effects on our health as ACE survivors. I typically help the ACE survivors with whom I work reduce their health risk by reducing their environmental exposure to potentially harmful substances in the three most common areas of

exposure—diet, personal care products, and their home environments.

I do this by helping them support and enhance liver function. I also help them cut out or significantly reduce dietary and environmental exposure to chemicals and other toxicants, such as polychlorinated biphenyls or PCBs, which are found in plastics and many types of seafood and have been strongly linked to HPA-axis dysregulation.[77] I also help address exposure to heavy metals, such as arsenic and mercury, which have been linked to depression,[78-79] anxiety,[79] behavioral changes,[78] and suicide risk.[79-80] By reducing our exposure to toxicants from dietary sources, in personal care products, and those to which we can be exposed in our home environments, we can decrease our risk for ACE-related chronic disease and experience improved health.

When we look at environmental factors, we also assess the use of substances such as alcohol and recreational drugs. This is important for us because, as ACE survivors, we are already at increased risk for decreases in our brain volume, and research demonstrates that as our lifetime alcohol intake increases, the amount of gray matter present in our brain decreases.[81] This research was conducted specifically on people who were not alcohol-dependent, suggesting that the decreases in brain volume were not due to alcoholism.

Interestingly, these results are not specific to alcohol use; instead, they apply to many other drugs as well. For example, adults who were nicotine-dependent[82] and those who used cannabis (marijuana) chronically were also found to have decreases in cortical gray matter.[83] Furthermore, individuals who smoked cannabis one to two times during adolescence were found to have decreases in brain gray matter volume, and after analyzing the data, researchers who conducted this study noted that it is most likely that the cannabis use led to the changes in brain structure, not the other way around.[84]

Because of the effects of psychoactive drugs on brain volume, I recommend that ACE survivors like us who are already at risk for these structural brain changes avoid the use of these substances as completely as possible. For those who have become dependent on the use of these substances, I make recommendations to help them address their dependence.

Diet-

The food we eat plays a significant role in whether or not we develop chronic disease, and I'd like to submit to you that this is even more true for ACE survivors like us. This is because of the effect of diet on the vagus nerve. I didn't always say this as decidedly as I'm about to say it now, but the evidence demonstrates, and I see time and time again with my patients, that in the long run, a well-balanced, low-fat, moderate-protein-containing, whole-foods, plant-based diet, coupled with ample water intake and supplemented with a high-quality source of plant-based omega-3 fatty acids and vitamins D and B_{12} where indicated, is most effective at preventing and/or reversing all four of the major categories of ACE-related chronic disease. For additional information on plant-based diets and why I recommend the supplements I do, see Appendix A.

So far we've discussed the vagus nerve as playing a crucial role in regulating inflammation levels via its inflammatory reflex, but what I didn't share is the fact that it also plays significant roles in regulating appetite, mood, heart rate, and more. Several studies demonstrate that consuming high-fat diets, such as the Ketogenic diet and standard American diet, for as few as one to

CHAPTER 8 FIND B.A.L.A.N.C.E.

seven days, induces inflammation within the vagus nerve system.[85] These types of diets also negatively impact vagal tone by compromising the nerve's ability to effectively communicate with the brain. This prevents the nerve from functioning as it should in maintaining optimal inflammation levels, a stable mood, healthy appetite, and modulating the stress response.

High-fat diets also have negative effects on the bacteria and other microbes in our gastrointestinal tracts. Researchers took a group of participants and studied them while consuming a plant-based diet, "rich in grains, legumes, fruits, and vegetables," and while consuming an animal-based diet composed of mainly meat, eggs, and cheese.[86] Each diet was consumed for five consecutive days. After the five days, study participants were observed for a six-day period. Participants consumed equal amounts of calories on the plant-based and animal-based diets.

At the end of the study, researchers found that participants had increased levels of bile-resistant bacteria while on the animal-based diet. This included high levels of *Bilophila wadsworthia*, a microbe that is known to cause an increase in gastrointestinal inflammation and that increases the risk for inflammatory bowel diseases like Crohn's disease and ulcerative colitis.

The results of this study demonstrate that in less than a week, the foods that we choose to consume can either serve as an additional stressor to our bodies, resulting in increased inflammation and a consequential worsening of mood and stress resiliency, or they can serve as a help to us along our healing journey, decreasing inflammation and helping to improve our moods, adaptability to stress, and overall wellbeing.

When I address diet with ACE survivors, I typically recommend that they implement an anti-inflammatory, phytonutrient-rich, minimally-processed, plant-based, 28-day elimination and challenge protocol, after which they reintroduce various foods into their diets and pay special attention to any changes that they notice in their pain levels, moods, energy levels, or other relevant areas of their health. My patients have found this exercise to be insightful because they learn so much about their bodies and are able to better determine which foods are best for maintaining the health of their unique bodies. It's also very effective in the long term because they see such great improvements in their health when they are able to choose foods based on this prized knowledge.

In addition to helping my patients determine which foods are best for their unique circumstances, I also make recommendations regarding when to eat for optimal health as an ACE survivor. For example, I typically recommend that the women with whom I work have two to three distinct meals per day and avoid snacking in between, as well as aim to end their last meal by or as close to 6 p.m. as possible. They then avoid eating again, including snacking and non-water beverages, until at least 12–14 hours later. This means that they typically have their breakfast around or after 6–8 a.m. the following morning.

Compared to six or more small meals per day and eating without respect to timing, this type of intermittent fasting has been shown to improve insulin sensitivity and fasting blood sugar levels.[87] It has also been shown to increase the overall lifespan,[88] and research suggests that it may even improve brain structure and function.[88]

Sleep-

Ensuring adequate quality and quantity of sleep is crucial for general wellbeing, but it is especially important for ACE survivors. This is because our circadian rhythms or internal clocks control the daily secretion of cortisol. Because of this intimate relationship between the circadian rhythm and the HPA axis, anything that disrupts the normal function of the circadian rhythm, such as disrupted or otherwise inadequate sleep, can negatively impact HPA-axis function.

Furthermore, there is also a very strong connection between sleep and inflammation, which we know is of great concern for ACE survivors. Poor sleep quality leads to an increase in inflammation and significantly elevates our risk for mental health concerns, reproductive concerns, autoimmune disorders, and metabolic syndrome. When a person is completely sleep-deprived, meaning that he or she does not sleep at all for two or more nights, we see immune system changes. This includes increases in inflammatory markers that are produced in the body whenever there is acute or chronic inflammation. We also see increases in inflammatory markers when a person is partially sleep-deprived, such as if he or she doesn't get enough sleep or has interrupted sleep for multiple nights.[89]

Because we are already at increased risk for having higher levels of inflammation as ACE survivors, and because inflammation drives all four major categories of ACE-related chronic disease, I typically recommend that the ACE survivors with whom I work aim for seven to nine hours of sleep each night, and for those who have a hard time falling or staying asleep at night, I make recommendations to regulate their circadian rhythms, address any anxiety or discomfort that may be preventing them from sleeping, or induce sleep at the appropriate time in order to help them achieve this goal.

Address Past Trauma

Through working with ACE survivors and doing my own internal work, I've come to realize that you can do all the things that improve physical health, but if you do not work through and emotionally process the events that took place in your childhood; if you hold on to anger, grief, self-pity, or any other negative emotion for extended periods of time; or if you completely avoid thinking or talking about your past in hopes that it will somehow disappear, then those negative emotions (even if they lie dormant and only surface when you are triggered by something external) will have negative effects on your health and potentially nullify all the work you are doing in the realm of your physical and mental health.

You see, if we leave elements of our past unaddressed, our negative emotions can actually activate our stress response and further disrupt our HPA-axis function as a result,[90] increasing our risk for chronic disease. Research also suggests that even if we limit the time spent thinking about these unresolved negative experiences that we've had, the emotions associated with the hurt can linger after we've stopped thinking about the incident(s) and continue to wreak havoc on our health.[91]

As an alternative to leaving the emotions associated with our past experiences unresolved, I recommend that ACE survivors make every effort to discuss their past experiences with those involved, if at all possible and if it is safe to do so. Research demonstrates that discussing situations in which we were hurt with those who have hurt us reduces anger and promotes forgiveness.[92] Anger is associated with increased activation of the stress response in many cases,[93] whereas forgiveness is associated with enhancements in tissue repair and immunity, decreases in anxiety and depression, and improvements in blood pressure, overall cardiovascular health, and longevity.[94]

Furthermore, in a study where researchers looked at participants' stress and forgiveness levels over their lifetimes, they found that while high stress levels were associated with worse mental and physical health, low levels of forgiveness were also associated with these negative outcomes. Interestingly, the research also demonstrated that those who experienced high stress levels but exhibited a high level of forgiveness had better health outcomes than those with high stress levels who were reluctant or less willing to forgive over their lifetimes.[95]

When Closure Isn't An Option-
While I believe it is extremely important to discuss our past so that we can come to this place of closure and forgiveness, I also understand that there are certain circumstances where discussing a situation may do more harm than good. This includes, among other circumstances, situations where offenders refuse to admit or take responsibility for their actions, situations where the offenders have passed away, and situations where the offender may pose a threat to you.

In cases like these, I've found cognitive behavioral therapy, also known as CBT, in combination with trauma-processing activities, to be a very valuable tool in the process of overcoming the emotional effects of adverse childhood experiences. In addition to helping to process and resolve feelings of guilt, anger, and powerlessness, as well as self-abuse, acting-out behavior, depression, anxiety, and other unwanted effects of ACEs, CBT has also been demonstrated to increase gray matter in the brain.[96–97] Trauma processing activities are beneficial because they help us to process our past experiences, address negative or otherwise unhealthy underlying beliefs and thought patterns, and counteract our ACE-induced, emotional barriers to healing. In my experience, CBT and trauma-processing activities are most effective when used together.

When I shared my story earlier, I mentioned that my biological father to date has never admitted to the fact that he was unfaithful to my mother during the 13 years that they were married and living together, despite the obvious, living, breathing evidence that he was. As you can imagine, this makes processing the situation and reconciliation difficult. Nonetheless, CBT-based and trauma-processing activities have been and continue to be extremely helpful to me when it comes to processing my emotions, modifying negative behaviors and reactions, and changing unhealthy thought patterns that I developed as a result of my reaction to my childhood experiences.

Normalize And/Or Optimize Hormones

Another important part of optimizing health as an ACE survivor in order to decrease risk for and improve or reverse the four major categories of ACE-related chronic disease is normalizing and/or optimizing hormones. This includes thyroid hormones, hormones that regulate blood sugar, HPA-axis hormones, reproductive hormones, and more.

In order to address thyroid function, I typically have my ACE survivors run several tests. While most primary care physicians usually check TSH as a screening test, I usually run, at bare minimum, TSH, free T3, free T4, and anti-thyroperoxidase and anti-thyroglobulin, both of which are antibodies and can indicate an autoimmune process in which your immune system is attacking your thyroid. My reason for running all five of these tests upfront is that it gives a more complete picture of thyroid function, compared to the TSH value alone.

This is especially important because, as I've shared, research demonstrates that the "normal" range for TSH is likely to be too high. This assertion is supported by the fact that, clinically, we see an increase in thyroid-related symptoms such as fatigue, mood changes, brain fog, and palpitations with suboptimal (yet technically "normal") thyroid function. We also see increased risk for chronic conditions such as mental health concerns,[98–100] reproductive concerns,[67, 101–103] other autoimmune diseases,[104] and metabolic concerns like diabetes,[105] cardiovascular disease,[106] and obesity[107] when thyroid function is suboptimal.

By running these tests and getting a more comprehensive view of what exactly is going on with the thyroid gland, I've been able to catch previously undiagnosed, early-stage thyroid disease in many patients and address their thyroid function before things escalate to the point of them needing to be put on thyroid hormone for the rest of their lives.

Each of the other hormones that we evaluate as a part of the B.A.L.A.N.C.E. Framework™ also has a significant effect on the health of ACE survivors. One of the hormones that we frequently assess and address is insulin.

We check insulin and blood sugar levels while in a fasting state in order to evaluate insulin sensitivity and glycemic control. We also look at cortisol levels, including the cortisol awakening response, or CAR, which is crucial for evaluating HPA-axis hypo- or hyper-reactivity and helps us uncover ACE-related causes of elevated inflammation levels, blood sugar dysregulation, autoimmune concerns, and mood and memory problems.

We look at reproductive hormones such as estrogen, progesterone, and their metabolites in order to evaluate and normalize these hormones for each woman's age and stage of life. We also look at other related hormones and markers. I use the information we gather from our objective testing to normalize and/or optimize hormone function using minimally invasive treatments and therapies.

Correct Gut Flora Abnormalities

As I've alluded to, we all have microbes that colonize our gastrointestinal tracts. These microbes can be bacteria, yeast, viruses, or other types. Some of them are normally found within our GI tracts and necessary for optimal health. Others should not be there and can cause harm to the body when present.

The composition of the microbes in your gut, also known as the microbiome, can have significant effects on your HPA axis, and this can influence your risk for ACE-related chronic disease. For example, your beneficial microbes are able to interact with your brain indirectly through the immune system and directly via your vagus nerve, which descends into your GI tract. Through a cascade of events, beneficial bacteria in the gut like *Lactobacillus rhamnosus*[108] and *Lactobacillus helveticus*[109] can help regulate HPA-axis function.

Not having enough beneficial microbes has the opposite effect. In fact, when we have insufficient amounts of beneficial bacteria or low microbial diversity in our GI tracts, this can result in hyperactivity of the HPA axis, difficulty adapting to stress in the short term, varying degrees of depression-like symptoms, depression, and other mood disorders in the long term, autoimmune diseases, and other conditions that are associated with HPA-axis dysregulation.[110] The most interesting part of this is the fact that abnormalities in our microbiomes can wreak havoc on our health without us experiencing gas, bloating, or any other gastrointestinal concerns.

When we experience traumatic events during childhood, it significantly impacts the composition and diversity of our microbiome. These changes to the microbiome frequently result in HPA-axis dysregulation.[111] In fact, research suggests that if you've experienced adversity at any point during your childhood, it is highly likely that, as an unwanted effect, you may be experiencing what we refer to as dysbiosis. Dysbiosis includes abnormal levels of beneficial microbes, high levels of non-beneficial or harmful microbes, and/or low levels of diversity as it relates to the various species of beneficial microbes that are present in your GI tract.

These unwanted dysbiotic changes that occur in response to ACEs can persist into adulthood, where they'll continue to negatively impact health if left unchecked. Additionally, because an imbalance of the microbiome can lead to inflammatory processes and HPA-axis activation,[110] your mood, ability to adapt to stressors, and risk for ACE-related chronic diseases can be negatively impacted by gastrointestinal dysbiosis and suboptimal GI health. On the other hand, restoring balance to the microbiome has been shown to significantly reduce many of the HPA-axis-related health problems we've discussed so far.

Because our gut bacteria can have such significant effects on our immune and nervous systems, and specifically the HPA axis, I recommend that many of the ACE survivors with whom I work run a test that provides us with detailed information about which microbes are present in their GI tracts, in what quantities, and how healthy their GI tracts are overall. From there, we make recommendations to reduce overall health risk and improve HPA-axis function. We do so by optimizing gastrointestinal function, reducing GI inflammation, and restoring balance to the microbiome.

Eliminate Or Reduce Medication

As a part of the B.A.L.A.N.C.E. Framework™, after we've put in the work necessary to support optimal health at the foundational level by addressing HPA-axis dysregulation, brain changes, and inflammation, and after we've begun to address the damage that has already been done to our health using minimally invasive modifications, the final step is to eliminate or reduce pharmaceutical medication. We do this by decreasing your need for medication first and then reducing or eliminating the medication itself. By supporting the body, giving it what it needs to function optimally, and then reducing the medication, we are able to limit the potential for unwanted side effects and withdrawal effects that come about when we try to discontinue certain pharmaceutical medication too quickly.

Regarding the process of discontinuing or tapering off medications, I only initiate this process with my patients in my private practice after we've laid the foundation for health, I've seen sufficient subjective and objective improvements in their health, and the patient and I collaboratively decide that it is a good time to begin the process.

I differentiate between discontinuing and tapering off medications because while some medications can be discontinued abruptly with minimal unwanted effects, the brain and body gradually compensate for the changes that other drugs impose upon it, and abrupt removal of those drugs does not allow the brain and body enough time to adjust to the changing concentrations of the medication. In most cases, this leads to unpleasant withdrawal symptoms.

To limit these unwanted effects, I help my patients discontinue medication that should be slowly tapered (such as psychotropic medications) using an incremental weaning protocol that takes into consideration factors such as how long the patient has been on the medication, the patient's current symptoms, genetics, and other factors that affect the rate at which a person can wean off of a medication. While weaning, I maintain close communication with my patients and support their health as indicated using natural therapies. Many of my patients have been able to decrease their medication dosage or discontinue their medication altogether using this approach.

B.A.L.A.N.C.E. Framework™ Summary

That was a brief overview of my B.A.L.A.N.C.E. Framework™, which I use to help ACE survivors like you and me overcome our predispositions to mental health concerns, hormonal or reproductive concerns, autoimmune disorders, and metabolic concerns. Because of the ACE-related changes that have taken place in our brains and bodies, we are at increased risk for these types of concerns, but this does not mean that we have to succumb to this increased risk. By using the elements of this framework, I have helped many ACE survivors preserve and restore optimal health. I believe that, by utilizing this framework, you can have similar results in your own life.

CHAPTER 9

DEAR THRIVER

....

Why ACEs don't have to define you, your future, or your dreams anymore

DEAR ACE-SURVIVING WOMAN,

Before I conclude this book, I want to write to you from my heart. I want to speak to you about the importance of us, as women, prioritizing our health for our own sakes, for the sakes of those who love us, and especially for the sake of our children, both living and unborn.

I'm a wife, mother, and working professional; I understand what it's like to be busy, just like I know you do. I know what it's like to feel overwhelmed. I know how easy it is to make a health or lifestyle choice that is convenient but not optimal. I know what it's like to feel like crying (and actually break down crying) because you are so overburdened with responsibilities you don't feel you'll be able to fulfill. I know what it's like to not have the time, energy, or motivation.

I know what it's like to feel powerless to change thought patterns, habits, and behaviors that you've nurtured for decades.

I know what it's like to experience changes in your life that you just don't feel ready to face. I know what it's like to wonder if you'll be able to raise healthy and emotionally resilient children. I know what it's like to look into the eyes of your children, see their innocence and beauty, and wish that you could give them the world. I know what it's like to question if you're doing what's best for them as their mother and to worry that you may have passed genetic predispositions and tendencies down to them that will be difficult to overcome.

I also know that, as women, we tend to feel the need to be strong for our families, current or future. And because I know these things, I want to reaffirm something that,

CHAPTER 9 DEAR THRIVER

deep down inside, you probably already know: as an ACE-surviving woman, the very best gift you can give to yourself and your family is the best and healthiest version of yourself.

Yes, your ACE history has impacted your present state of physical and mental health and the health of your relationships. Yes, your traumatic upbringing has affected your past. It may have even affected your children's past. However, please hear me out on this one; it does not have to affect your future.

You can choose today to prioritize your physical, mental, spiritual, and social health and become the best version of yourself.

Remember my mom's story? She *chose* to overcome the trauma she had experienced and its effects on her life. Yes, my siblings and I were affected by our early upbringing, but seeing our mother overcome the things she overcame did something for us. Seeing my mother's determination, grit, resolve, and perseverance helped me begin to develop and cultivate those traits and capabilities as well. Despite the fact that I had experienced ACEs, my mother's choices inspired me. They motivated me to overcome the effects of the trauma I had experienced in my own life. I learned resilience from her.

And in case our story isn't enough, here's what the research in the realm of behavioral health says: Although experiencing one or more ACEs is associated with poorer mental health, this association dissipates in the context of high resilience. In other words, if you or your children have experienced ACEs and also have low levels of resilience, then you are at increased risk for poor mental health, but—here's the good part—if you have experienced one or more ACEs but you've learned resilience, you are no more likely to have poor mental health than a person who has not experienced any ACEs.[112]

This is why I'm so passionate about teaching women to become physically and emotionally resilient. When we learn resilience, we're able to confer that resilience to our children and, in doing so, we can help them mitigate their own risk. *But…* it's hard to be resilient when you don't feel well, which is why I encourage you to use my B.A.L.A.N.C.E. Framework™ to address the foundational changes that took place in your body and brain during childhood. Use it to help yourself address the damage that's already been done in the form of your ACE-related health diagnoses.

We've got to work on your physical and mental health first, then we've got to make sure that you're actively processing your past experiences in a healthy manner and learning new skills and coping mechanisms. This is how you can become the very best version of yourself for yourself, your significant other, others who love you, and especially those precious children that you have or will have.

From one ACE-surviving woman to another: I'm happy to know that you've survived your early environment; we don't all survive. I'm proud of the progress you've made in your life so far. I appeal to you: please, continue to progress. Don't allow the cycle to be perpetuated in your life. You owe it to yourself first, but also to your significant other and to your children, to prioritize and optimize your health so that you can live life on your own terms, raise physically healthy and emotionally resilient children, and rise above your past and present circumstances.

As a woman who has experienced ACEs and now has two precious, beautiful, and innocent children who look to me for their every need, my mission is to help as many ACE-surviving women as possible achieve optimal health and, by doing so, help them to break the cycle in their own lives so that both they and their families can live their healthiest and best lives each day.

I'd like to help you do the same.

DR. JANELLE LOUIS, ND

APPENDIX A:
Explanation of My Dietary Recommendations

WHEN IT COMES TO diet, I typically recommend moderate intake of complex carbohydrates (50- 60% of caloric intake), ample intake of preferably plant-based protein (15-20% of total caloric intake), and comparatively low fat intake (about 30% of total caloric intake).

These recommendations are based on my analysis of an inordinate amount of research; nevertheless, the results of one particular landmark prospective study summarize the conclusions I've drawn. This study found that both low- and high-carbohydrate containing diets are associated with increased all-cause mortality, compared to moderate-carbohydrate-containing diets. In other words, those who habitually consumed diets in which less than 40% or greater than 70% of energy came from carbohydrates were more likely to die from all causes combined, compared to those who consumed diets where 50-55% of caloric intake came from carbohydrates. To put it simply, moderate consumption of carbohydrates appears to be associated with increased longevity.

That 15,428-person study also found that diets based on "animal-derived protein and fat sources, from sources such as lamb, beef, pork, and chicken, were associated with higher mortality, whereas those that favoured [*sic*] plant-derived protein and fat intake, from sources such as vegetables, nuts, peanut butter, and whole-grain breads, were associated with lower mortality."[113]

These results suggest that the source of food—where you get your proteins and fats—may modify the association between carbohydrate intake and mortality. Again, to put it more simply, it appears that even if you eat a diet that is higher or lower in carbohydrates than the suggested moderate intake, you may be able to increase your likelihood of longevity by replacing animal-based sources of proteins and fats with plant-based sources.

My Professional Opinion of Plant-Based Diets

My professional opinion of plant-based diets that consist of whole, minimally processed foods aligns with the official position of the Academy of Nutrition and Dietetics. They expressed the conclusion of my research well when they stated that "appropriately planned vegetarian, including vegan, diets are healthful, nutritionally adequate, and may provide health benefits for the prevention and treatment of certain diseases. These diets are appropriate for all stages of the life cycle, including pregnancy, lactation, infancy, childhood, adolescence, older adulthood, and for athletes."[114]

Because we are at increased risk for over 30 different chronic diseases as ACE-surviving women, plant-based diets offer health benefits that (if we're really thinking about and being proactive concerning our health) we cannot easily refuse.

The Academy of Nutrition and Dietetics continued on to report that "low intake of saturated fat and high intakes of vegetables, fruits, whole grains, legumes, soy products, nuts, and seeds (all rich in fiber and phytochemicals) are characteristics of vegetarian and vegan diets that produce lower total and low-density lipoprotein cholesterol levels and better serum glucose control. These factors contribute to reduction of chronic disease."[114]

Potential Nutrient Deficiencies

In spite of this statement from the world's largest organization of food and nutrition professionals, we're all entitled to our own opinions, and this is one of the reasons why there is still some controversy regarding the therapeutic use of plant-based diets. Throughout my career, I've been the type of person who is determined to find the facts, the high-quality scientific data, and draw my conclusions from them. As a result, I've done an immense amount of research into various patterns of eating and I've seen the effects of each of them in my clinical practice.

I welcome you to do your own research because I'm confident that, if you come to the science with an open mind, you'll come to the same conclusions that I have. Nevertheless, if you would like for me to spare you the time and energy, I'll share information regarding what I believe will be your most pressing questions regarding this way of eating. I'm assuming you, like many of my patients, want to know whether or not there is a risk of nutrient deficiency with consumption of a plant-based diet and whether or not you should be supplementing any nutrients while consuming a balanced, whole-foods, minimally-processed, low-fat, moderate-protein-containing, plant-based diet. I'll use the remainder of this appendix to answer these questions.

Protein- The United States Department of Agriculture recommends that individuals above the age of 19 consume at least 0.8 grams of protein per kilogram of body weight per day. According to these guidelines, a person who weighs 125 pounds should consume at least 45 grams of protein per day, while a person who weighs 165 pounds should consume at least 60 grams of protein per day.

For perspective, one cup of cooked lentils contains about 18 grams of protein and a half-cup of almonds contains about 15 grams of protein. One large baked potato and a cup of cooked green peas contain about 16 grams of protein.[115] That's almost half the recommended daily protein intake for a 125-pound person and almost one-third of the recommended daily protein intake for a 165-pound person. Needless the say, protein deficiency is not a real concern on plant-based diets in developed countries where sufficient food is both available and accessible.

You may have also heard the narrative that plant-based proteins are somehow inferior to animal-based proteins because they are "incomplete proteins," whereas animal products are "complete proteins." Well, while it is true that aside from quinoa, soy, and a few other food items, plant-based foods typically do not contain all of the essential amino acids (which our bodies can't make and we must get from food), it's also true that you do not need to consume all of the essential amino acids in one meal in order to avoid deficiency. In other words, there is no need for protein pairing as was previously recommended and, as long as we consume ample calories and a variety of different plant-based foods each day, there is no risk of amino acid or protein deficiency.

Legumes and Grains- Many people express concern about lectins (also known as phytohemagglutinins), phytic acid, enzyme inhibitors, and other anti-nutrients preventing the absorption of their nutrients if they eat legumes or grains. However, as long as we are cooking our beans and grains before eating them, the concern regarding dietary anti-nutrients is also a non-issue. Research demonstrates that boiling soybeans in water for as little as 5-10 minutes virtually eliminated all lectin activity.[116-118] Phytic acid, which is typically found in both grains and legumes, are also made significantly less active by cooking, boiling, sprouting, or leavening such as in baking leavened bread.[119-120] Additionally, enzyme inhibitors are made significantly less active by cooking, boiling, or sprouting,[119] and chronic ingestion of residual levels is unlikely to pose risks to human health.[121]

***Iron and Zinc*-** While people who avoid meat often have lower ferritin levels than omnivores despite the fact that the total iron intake between the two groups is comparable, the differences between hemoglobin levels in the two groups are small and are rarely associated with anemia.[122] There aren't very many high-quality studies on objectively observable zinc deficiency as marked by low serum zinc concentrations in people avoiding meat, but the data we do have suggest no difference in zinc concentrations of omnivores and children and adults avoiding meat.[123] There is some evidence that adolescents who avoid meat may have lower zinc concentrations than adolescent omnivores, however, researchers noted that the data is particularly conflicting because many studies look at data from individuals living in or who have recently migrated from underdeveloped nations, and these people may be predisposed to iron and zinc deficiency because of non-dietary factors, such as chronic inflammation, parasitic infections, overweight, and genetic hemoglobin disorders.[122]

Calcium- Evidence suggests that adherents to high-fat diets such as the standard American and Ketogenic diets are at increased risk for osteoporosis and fractures. This is likely due to the highly acidic nature of the diet. Researchers believe that plant-based adherents do not exhibit increased risk of osteoporosis because of their diets' low acid load. Low acid load is correlated with lower bone resorption, higher bone mineral density, and higher intake of potassium-rich foods such as fruits and vegetables. Studies show that the acid load in plant-based diets is either minimal or completely absent, while the omnivorous standard American diet tends to produce 50 to 70 mEq of acid per day. The low acid content of plant-based diets protects those who eat them from osteoporosis and fractures.[124]

The Need For Supplementation

Now that I've touched on the most common arguments against plant-based diets, I'll share why I recommend supplementing with omega-3 fatty acids and vitamins D and B_{12}. I'll start with omega-3s, which will require a bit of background information, and then I'll briefly discuss vitamin D and vitamin B_{12}.

Omega-3 Fatty Acids

First of all, omega-3 fatty acids have anti-inflammatory effects on the body.[125] The three most important omega-3 fatty acids in human physiology are alpha-linolenic acid (ALA), eicosapentaenoic acid (EPA), and docosahexaenoic acid (DHA). ALA is mostly found in plant-based foods like walnuts and flax seeds and is converted in the body to EPA and DHA. The body's process of making EPA and DHA from ALA is limited to 8-20% for conversion of ALA to EPA and 1-9% for the conversion of ALA to DHA.[126-127] Outside of this conversion, EPA and DHA are mostly found in fatty fish and certain species of algae.

Arachidonic acid (ARA), on the other hand, is a polyunsaturated omega-6 fatty acid that plays a crucial role in the body's signaling for pain and inflammation.[128] Our bodies make very small amounts of ARA from linoleic acid,[129-130] a shorter omega-6 fatty acid found in nuts, seeds, and their oils, but we get the vast majority of ARA from our diets when we consume animal products such as fish, chicken, beef, pork, other meat, eggs, cheese, and dairy. ARA has a mostly pro-inflammatory effect on the body.

When we eat foods that contain pre-formed ARA, the pro-inflammatory ARA competes with anti-inflammatory omega-3 fatty acids to bind to certain enzymes.[129] When ARA succeeds in binding to the appropriate enzyme, the body begins to produce more pro-inflammatory metabolites like prostaglandins, and this leads to increased inflammation within the body. To limit the pro-inflammatory effects of ARA on the body, which we know are detrimental to us as ACE survivors, it's crucial that we decrease our intake of pre-formed ARA and increase our intake of omega-3 fatty acids.

This is because, when it comes to omega-6 and omega-3 fatty acids, the ratio of omega-6s to omega-3s is more important than the actual amount that we consume of each fatty acid type. While the ideal omega-6 to omega-3 ratio is 4 to 1 or lower, some estimates report that the ratio in the standard American diet may be anywhere from 15:1 to 16.7:1.[131]

While those who consume diets that are rich in pre-formed ARA need large amounts of dietary omega-3 fatty acids to counteract its effect, those who eat mostly plant-based diets don't need to consume as much omega-3 fatty acids. Again, this is because their dietary intake of pre-formed ARA is so low and the ratio is what's most important for optimal inflammation levels and overall wellness, not the absolute amounts.

In other words, although plant-based diets are lower in both pro-inflammatory ARA and in anti-inflammatory omega-3 fatty acids than omnivorous diets, those who avoid dietary consumption of fish, poultry, and other meat do not exhibit clinical signs of omega-3 deficiency.[132] This is in spite of their very low or virtually absent intake of EPA and DHA. Again we see that the omega-6 to omega-3 ratio is more important than the absolute amount that we consume of each.

I typically recommend that anyone who consumes a plant-based diet consume about 4 grams of ALA per day, the equivalent of less than two tablespoons of flaxseeds.[133] This dosage more than doubles the National Academy of Medicine's adequate intake value[134] for males and for women in all phases of life, including women of childbearing age and women who are pregnant, breastfeeding, or menopausal.

Alternatively, I frequently recommend taking a high-quality, plant-based (algae) omega-3 supplement containing at least 200-300 mg per day of EPA and DHA. Research shows that individuals on a plant-based diet who make this change respond well to these relatively low doses of supplemental omega-3s. They are able to benefit from the omega-3s in the algae oil[132] while avoiding the increased cardiovascular and other health risks due to heavy metals like arsenic and mercury in fish; the increased neurological, immunological, and reproductive risk associated with increased body burden from chemicals such as polychlorinated biphenyls and other endocrine-disrupting compounds frequently found in fish;[135-136] and the overabundance of pre-formed, pro-inflammatory ARA found in other animal-based products.

Vitamin D

When it comes to vitamin D, our dietary sources are mainly limited to fish liver oils, fatty fish, egg yolks, and fortified milks and cereals. Research demonstrates that most of the population is either insufficient or deficient in vitamin D, whether they consume a plant-based or an omnivorous diet. To be more precise, 77% of Americans have vitamin D levels below 30 ng/ mL, indicating that only 23% of Americans have vitamin D levels within the "normal" range.[137] This is why I typically recommend that everyone have their vitamin D levels checked and supplement if needed in order to achieve and maintain optimal levels. This is regardless of the type of diet consumed.

Vitamin B_{12}

Now when it comes to vitamin B_{12}, neither plants nor animals make B_{12}; it's actually made by bacteria. Animals consume bacteria, humans eat meat from these animals, and that's mostly how omnivores get their B_{12}. Those who consume plant-based diets get dietary vitamin B_{12} from fortified foods. Although B_{12} is a water-soluble vitamin, our bodies are able to store it in the liver for long periods of time. In fact, if you were to stop consuming all sources of B_{12} today, you would still have enough stored up to last you 3-5 years.[138]

Vitamin B12 is extremely important to health because deficiencies can lead to elevations in an amino acid called homocysteine, which leads to increased inflammation, neurological concerns, cardiovascular concerns, and all of the complications that come along with them. In order to avoid deficiency and help keep homocysteine levels optimal, I typically recommend supplementing with vitamin B12 on a healthy, balanced, plant-based diet. Because the body limits how much B12 can be absorbed from the gastrointestinal tract at a time, I specifically recommend taking this vitamin in divided doses (e.g. with 2 distinct meals several hours apart) whenever possible. This maximizes absorption of the vitamin and makes it more likely that you will achieve your daily requirements.

Final Thoughts Regarding Optimal Food Choices For ACE Survivors

Understanding the ins-and-outs of what to eat can be confusing in today's world, especially when there are so many industries that are self-serving and otherwise financially driven. With many of these big industries funding "scientific" studies that are little more than propaganda, it's now possible to find research that supports almost any viewpoint. This is why it's so important for us to be able to differentiate between high- and low-quality research and to draw conclusions based on reliable, scientific facts and not conjecture. When we learn to come to the research with an open mind and a critical eye and adjust our habits based on our findings, we'll be better able to be our own health advocates, and we'll be better equipped to take back control into our own hands so that we can live our healthiest—physically, mentally, emotionally, spiritually, and socially—and best lives on our own terms.

REFERENCES

1. Cortisol: What It Does & How To Regulate Cortisol Levels. WebMD. https://www.webmd.com/a-to-z-guides/what-is-cortisol#1.
2. Negative Feedback Regulation of Hormone Release in the Hypothalamic-Pituitary Axis. University of Washington Courses. https://courses.washington.edu/conj/bess/feedback/newfeedback.html. Accessed April 19, 2019.
3. van Bodegom M, Homberg JR, Henckens MJAG. Modulation of the Hypothalamic-Pituitary-Adrenal Axis by Early Life Stress Exposure. *Front Cell Neurosci*. 2017;11:87. Published 2017 Apr 19. doi:10.3389/fncel.2017.00087
4. Dube SR, Fairweather D, Pearson WS, Felitti VJ, Anda RF, Croft JB. Cumulative childhood stress and autoimmune diseases in adults. *Psychosom Med*. 2009;71(2):243-50. doi: 10.1097/PSY.0b013e3181907888
5. Vreeburg SA, Hoogendijk WJG, van Pelt J, et al. Major Depressive Disorder and Hypothalamic-Pituitary-Adrenal Axis Activity: Results From a Large Cohort Study. *Arch Gen Psychiatry*. 2009;66(6):617–626. doi:10.1001/archgenpsychiatry.2009.50
6. Danese A, Pariante CM, Caspi A, Taylor A, Poulton R. Childhood maltreatment predicts adult inflammation in a life-course study. *Proc Natl Acad Sci U S A*. 2007;104(4):1319-24. Published 2007 Jan 17. doi: 10.1073/pnas.0610362104
7. About the CDC-Kaiser ACE Study |Violence Prevention|Injury Center|CDC. Centers for Disease Control and Prevention. https://www.cdc.gov/violenceprevention/childabuseandneglect/acestudy/about.html. Accessed April 19, 2019.

8. Kessler RC, McLaughlin KA, Green JG, et al. Childhood adversities and adult psychopathology in the WHO World Mental Health Surveys. *Br J Psychiatry.* 2010;197(5):378–385. doi:10.1192/bjp.bp.110.080499

9. Lyra E Silva NM, Lam MP, Soares CN, et al. Insulin Resistance as a Shared Pathogenic Mechanism Between Depression and Type 2 Diabetes. *Front Psychiatry.* 2019;10:57. doi:10.3389/fpsyt.2019.00057

10. Anwer T, Sharma M, Pillai KK, et al. Effect of Withania somnifera on insulin sensitivity in non-insulin-dependent diabetes mellitus rats. *Basic Clin Pharmacol Toxicol.* 2008;102(6):498-503. doi:10.1111/j.1742-7843.2008.00223.x

11. Udayakumar R, Kasthurirengan S, Mariashibu TS, et al. Hypoglycaemic and hypolipidaemic effects of Withania somnifera root and leaf extracts on alloxan-induced diabetic rats. *Int J Mol Sci.* 2009;10(5):2367–82. doi:10.3390/ijms10052367

12. Chandrasekhar K, Kapoor J, Anishetty S. A prospective, randomized double-blind, placebo-controlled study of safety and efficacy of a high-concentration full-spectrum extract of ashwagandha root in reducing stress and anxiety in adults. *Indian J Psychol Med.* 2012;34(3):255–62. doi:10.4103/0253-7176.106022

13. de Punder K, Entringer S, Heim C, et al. Inflammatory Measures in Depressed Patients With and Without a History of Adverse Childhood Experiences. *Front Psychiatry.* 2018;9:610. doi:10.3389/fpsyt.2018.00610

14. Sheridan MA, Fox NA, Zeanah CH, et al. Variation in neural development as a result of exposure to institutionalization early in childhood. *Proc Natl Acad Sci U S A.* 2012;109(32):12927–32. doi:10.1073/pnas.1200041109

15. Haier RJ, Jung RE, Yeo RA, et al. Structural brain variation and general intelligence. *Neuroimage.* 2004;23(1):425-33. doi:10.1016/j.neuroimage.2004.04.025

16. Luby JL, Belden AC, Jackson JJ, et al. Early Childhood Depression and Alterations in the Trajectory of Gray Matter Maturation in Middle Childhood and Early Adolescence. *JAMA Psychiatry.* 2016;73(1):31–38. doi:10.1001/jamapsychiatry.2015.2356

17. Chapman DP, Whitfield CL, Felitti VJ, et al. Adverse childhood experiences and the risk of depressive disorders in adulthood. J Affect Disord. 2004;82(2):217-25. doi:10.1016/j.jad.2003.12.013

18. Sareen J, Henriksen CA, Bolton SL, et al. Adverse childhood experiences in relation to mood and anxiety disorders in a population-based sample of active military personnel. *Psychol Med.* 2013;43(1):73-84. doi:10.1017/S003329171200102X.

19. Choi NG, DiNitto DM, Marti CN, et al. Association of adverse childhood experiences with lifetime mental and substance use disorders among men and women aged 50+ years. *Int Psychogeriatr.* 2017;29(3):359-72. doi: 10.1017/S1041610216001800.

20. Aas M, Henry C, Andreassen OA, et al. The role of childhood trauma in bipolar disorders. *Int J Bipolar Disord.* 2016;4(1):2. doi:10.1186/s40345-015-0042-0

21. Varese F, Smeets F, Drukker M, et al. Childhood adversities increase the risk of psychosis: a meta-analysis of patient-control, prospective- and cross-sectional cohort studies. *Schizophr Bull.* 2012;38(4):661–671. doi:10.1093/schbul/sbs050

22. Felitti VJ, Anda RF, Nordenberg D, et al. Relationship of childhood abuse and household dysfunction to many of the leading causes of death in adults. The Adverse Childhood Experiences (ACE) Study. *Am J Prev Med.* 1998;14(4):245-58.

23. Dube SR, Anda RF, Felitti VJ, et al. Childhood abuse, household dysfunction, and the risk of attempted suicide throughout the life span: findings from the Adverse Childhood Experiences Study. *JAMA.* 2001;286(24):3089-96.

24. Cheong EV, Sinnott C, Dahly D, et al. Adverse childhood experiences (ACEs) and later-life depression: perceived social support as a potential protective factor. *BMJ Open* 2017;7:e013228. doi: 10.1136/bmjopen-2016-013228

25. Dube SR, Anda RF, Whitfield CL, et al. Long-term consequences of childhood sexual abuse by gender of victim. *Am J Prev Med.* 2005;28(5):430-8. doi:10.1016/j.amepre.2005.01.015

26. Dube SR, Anda RF, Felitti VJ, et al. Adverse childhood experiences and personal alcohol abuse as an adult. *Addict Behav.* 2002;27(5):713-25.

27. Dube SR, Felitti VJ, Dong M, et al. Childhood abuse, neglect, and household dysfunction and the risk of illicit drug use: the adverse childhood experiences study. *Pediatrics*. 2003;111(3):564-72.

28. Whitfield CL, Dube SR, Felitti VJ, et al. Adverse childhood experiences and hallucinations. Child Abuse Negl. 2005;29(7):797-810. doi:10.1016/j.chiabu.2005.01.004

29. Anda RF, Brown DW, Felitti VJ, et al. Adverse childhood experiences and prescribed psychotropic medications in adults. *Am J Prev Med*. 2007;32(5):389–394. doi:10.1016/j.amepre.2007.01.005

30. Rush AJ, Trivedi MH, Wisniewski SR, et al. Acute and longer-term outcomes in depressed outpatients requiring one or several treatment steps: a STAR*D report. Am J Psychiatry. 2006;163(11):1905-17. doi:10.1176/ajp.2006.163.11.1905

31. De Vera MA, Bérard A. Antidepressant use during pregnancy and the risk of pregnancy-induced hypertension. *Br J Clin Pharmacol*. 2012;74(2):362–369. doi:10.1111/j.1365-2125.2012.04196.x

32. Liu X, Agerbo E, Ingstrup KG, et al. Antidepressant use during pregnancy and psychiatric disorders in offspring: Danish nationwide register based cohort study. *BMJ* 2017;358:j3668. doi:10.1136/bmj.j3668

33. Gramaglia C, Gambaro E, Bartolomei G, et al. Increased Risk of Metabolic Syndrome in Antidepressants Users: A Mini Review. *Front Psychiatry*. 2018;9:621. doi:10.3389/fpsyt.2018.00621

34. Pramyothin P, Khaodhiar L. Metabolic syndrome with the atypical antipsychotics. *Curr Opin Endocrinol Diabetes Obes*. 2010;17(5):460-6. doi:10.1097/MED.0b013e32833de61c

35. DuPont RL. "Should Patients With Substance Use Disorders Be Prescribed Benzodiazepines?" No. *J Addict Med*. 2017;11(2):84-6. doi:10.1097/ADM.0000000000000291.

36. Magiakou MA, Mastorakos G, Webster E, et al. The hypothalamic-pituitary-adrenal axis and the female reproductive system. *Ann N Y Acad Sci*. 1997;816:42-56.

37. Smith MV, Gotman N, Yonkers KA. Early Childhood Adversity and Pregnancy Outcomes. *Matern Child Health J*. 2016;20(4):790–798. doi:10.1007/s10995-015-1909-5

38. Chung EK, Nurmohamed L, Mathew L, Elo IT, Coyne JC, Culhane JF. Risky health behaviors among mothers-to-be: the impact of adverse childhood experiences. *Acad Pediatr.* 2010;10(4):245–251. doi:10.1016/j.acap.2010.04.003

39. Hillis SD, Anda RF, Dube SR, et al. The association between adverse childhood experiences and adolescent pregnancy, long-term psychosocial consequences, and fetal death. *Pediatrics.* 2004;113(2):320-7.

40. Möhler E, Matheis V, Marysko M, et al. Complications during pregnancy, peri- and postnatal period in a sample of women with a history of child abuse. *J Psychosom Obstet Gynaecol.* 2008;29(3):193-8. doi: 10.1080/01674820801934252

41. Jacobs MB, Boynton-Jarrett RD, Harville EW. Adverse childhood event experiences, fertility difficulties and menstrual cycle characteristics. *J Psychosom Obstet Gynaecol.* 2015;36(2):46–57. doi:10.3109/0167482X.2015.1026892

42. Farber EW, Herbert SE, Reviere SL. Childhood abuse and suicidality in obstetrics patients in a hospital-based urban prenatal clinic. Gen Hosp Psychiatry. 1996;18(1):56-60.

43. Hollingsworth K, Callaway L, Duhig M, Matheson S, Scott J. The association between maltreatment in childhood and pre-pregnancy obesity in women attending an antenatal clinic in Australia. *PLoS One.* 2012;7(12):e51868. doi:10.1371/journal.pone.0051868

44. Boynton-Jarrett R, Rich-Edwards JW, Jun HJ, et al. Abuse in childhood and risk of uterine leiomyoma: the role of emotional support in biologic resilience. *Epidemiology.* 2011;22(1):6–14. doi:10.1097/EDE.0b013e3181ffb172

45. Bertone-Johnson ER, Whitcomb BW, Missmer SA, et al. Early life emotional, physical, and sexual abuse and the development of premenstrual syndrome: a longitudinal study. *J Womens Health (Larchmt).* 2014;23(9):729–739. doi:10.1089/jwh.2013.4674

46. Lukasse M, Vangen S, Øian P, et al. Childhood abuse and caesarean section among primiparous women in the Norwegian Mother and Child Cohort Study. *BJOG.* 2010;117(9):1153-7. doi: 10.1111/j.1471-0528.2010.02627.x.

47. Pyykönen A, Gissler M, Løkkegaard E, et al. Cesarean section trends in the Nordic Countries - a comparative analysis with the Robson classification. *Acta Obstet Gynecol Scand.* 2017;96(5):607-16. doi: 10.1111/aogs.13108.

48. FastStats - Births - Method of Delivery. Centers for Disease Control and Prevention. https://www.cdc.gov/nchs/fastats/delivery.htm. Accessed April 22, 2019.
49. Fertility Factors. Oregon Health & Science University. https://www.ohsu.edu/xd/health/services/women/services/fertility/fertility-services/evaulation-for-fertility/fertility-factors.cfm. Accessed April 22, 2019.
50. Women & Autoimmunity. AARDA. https://www.aarda.org/who-we-help/patients/women-and-autoimmunity/#1481574903922-68688035-6be6. Accessed April 22, 2019.
51. Pavlov VA, Tracey KJ. The vagus nerve and the inflammatory reflex--linking immunity and metabolism. *Nat Rev Endocrinol*. 2012;8(12):743–754. doi:10.1038/nrendo.2012.189
52. Song H, Fang F, Tomasson G, et al. Association of Stress-Related Disorders With Subsequent Autoimmune Disease. *JAMA*. 2018;319(23):2388-400. doi: 10.1001/jama.2018.7028.
53. Stojanovich L, Marisavljevich D. Stress as a trigger of autoimmune disease. *Autoimmun Rev.* 2008;7(3):209-13. doi:10.1016/j.autrev.2007.11.007.
54. Black PH. The inflammatory response is an integral part of the stress response: Implications for atherosclerosis, insulin resistance, type II diabetes and metabolic syndrome X. *Brain Behav Immun*. 2003;17(5):350-64.
55. Brody B. Atherosclerosis: Your Arteries Age by Age. WebMD. https://www.webmd.com/heart-disease/features/atherosclerosis-your-arteries-age-by-age. Accessed April 22, 2019.
56. Pierce JB, Kershaw KN, Kiefe CI, et al. Abstract 14977: Association of Childhood Psychosocial Environment With Incident Cardiovascular Disease in Middle Adulthood: The Coronary Artery Risk Development in Young Adults (CARDIA) Study. 2018;138,No. Suppl_1.
57. Su S, Wang X, Pollock JS, et al. Adverse childhood experiences and blood pressure trajectories from childhood to young adulthood: the Georgia stress and Heart study. *Circulation*. 2015;131(19):1674–1681. doi:10.1161/CIRCULATIONAHA.114.013104.
58. Huffhines L, Noser A, Patton SR. The Link Between Adverse Childhood Experiences and Diabetes. *Curr Diab Rep*. 2016;16(6):54. doi:10.1007/s11892-016-0740-8

59. Fuemmeler BF, Dedert E, McClernon FJ, Beckham JC. Adverse childhood events are associated with obesity and disordered eating: results from a U.S. population-based survey of young adults. *J Trauma Stress.* 2009;22(4):329–333. doi:10.1002/jts.20421

60. Isohookana R, Marttunen M, Hakko H, et al. The impact of adverse childhood experiences on obesity and unhealthy weight control behaviors among adolescents. Compr Psychiatry. 2016;71:17-24. doi: 10.1016/j.comppsych.2016.08.002.

61. Su S, Wang X, Pollock JS, et al. Adverse childhood experiences and blood pressure trajectories from childhood to young adulthood: the Georgia stress and Heart study. *Circulation.* 2015;131(19):1674–1681. doi:10.1161/CIRCULATIONAHA.114.013104

62. Anda RF, Felitti VJ, Bremner JD, et al. The enduring effects of abuse and related adverse experiences in childhood. A convergence of evidence from neurobiology and epidemiology. *Eur Arch Psychiatry Clin Neurosci.* 2005;256(3):174–186. doi:10.1007/s00406-005-0624-4

63. Deschênes SS, Graham E, Kivimäki M, et al. Adverse Childhood Experiences and the Risk of Diabetes: Examining the Roles of Depressive Symptoms and Cardiometabolic Dysregulations in the Whitehall II Cohort Study. Diabetes Care. 2018;41(10):2120-6. doi: 10.2337/dc18-0932.

64. Ramaswamy K, Masand PS, Nasrallah HA. Do certain atypical antipsychotics increase the risk of diabetes: a critical review of 17 pharmacoepidemiologic studies. 2006. In: Database of Abstracts of Reviews of Effects (DARE): Quality-assessed Reviews [Internet]. York (UK): Centre for Reviews and Dissemination (UK); 1995-. Available from: https://www.ncbi.nlm.nih.gov/books/NBK72408/

65. Beyazyüz M, Albayrak Y, Eğilmez OB, Albayrak N, Beyazyüz E. Relationship between SSRIs and Metabolic Syndrome Abnormalities in Patients with Generalized Anxiety Disorder: A Prospective Study. *Psychiatry Investig.* 2013;10(2):148–154. doi:10.4306/pi.2013.10.2.148

66. Spencer CA, Hollowell JG, Kazarosyan M, et al. National Health and Nutrition Examination Survey III thyroid-stimulating hormone (TSH)-thyroperoxidase antibody relationships demonstrate that TSH upper reference limits may be skewed by occult thyroid dysfunction. J Clin Endocrinol Metab. 2007;92(11):4236-40.

67. Sordia-Hernandez LH, Morales Martinez A, Gris JM, et al. Normal "high" thyroid stimulating hormone (TSH) levels and pregnancy rates in patients undergoing IVF with donor eggs. Clin Exp Obstet Gynecol. 2014;41(5):517-20.

68. Ising M, Depping AM, Siebertz A, et al. Polymorphisms in the FKBP5 gene region modulate recovery from psychosocial stress in healthy controls. Eur J Neurosci. 2008;28(2):389-98. doi: 10.1111/j.1460-9568.2008.06332.x.

69. Kassi E, Nasiri-Ansari N, Spilioti E, et al. Vitamin D interferes with glucocorticoid responsiveness in human peripheral blood mononuclear target cells. Cell Mol Life Sci. 2016;73(22):4341-54. doi:10.1007/s00018-016-2281-3

70. Monteleone P, Maj M, Beinat L, et al. Blunting by chronic phosphatidylserine administration of the stress-induced activation of the hypothalamo-pituitary-adrenal axis in healthy men. Eur J Clin Pharmacol. 1992;42(4):385-8.

71. Monteleone P, Beinat L, Tanzillo C, et al. Effects of phosphatidylserine on the neuroendocrine response to physical stress in humans. Neuroendocrinology. 1990;52(3):243-8. doi:10.1159/000125593

72. Hunter MR, Gillespie BW, Chen SY. Urban Nature Experiences Reduce Stress in the Context of Daily Life Based on Salivary Biomarkers. 2019;10:722. doi:10.3389/fpsyg.2019.00722

73. Im SG, Choi H, Jeon YH, et al. Comparison of Effect of Two-Hour Exposure to Forest and Urban Environments on Cytokine, Anti-Oxidant, and Stress Levels in Young Adults. *Int J Environ Res Public Health*. 2016;13(7):625. doi:10.3390/ijerph13070625

74. Yeager R, Riggs DW, DeJarnett N, et al. Association Between Residential Greenness and Cardiovascular Disease Risk. JAHA. 2018;7(24) doi:10.1161/JAHA.118.009117.

75. Colcombe SJ, Erickson KI, Scalf PE, et al. Aerobic exercise training increases brain volume in aging humans. J Gerontol A Biol Sci Med Sci. 2006;61(11):1166-70.

76. Liu PZ, Nusslock R. Exercise-Mediated Neurogenesis in the Hippocampus via BDNF. *Front Neurosci*. 2018;12:52. Published 2018 Feb 7. doi:10.3389/fnins.2018.00052

REFERENCES

77. Zimmer K. Effects of persistent environmental pollutants on the HPA-axis. *Acta Vet Scand*. 2012;54(Suppl 1):S17. Published 2012 Feb 24. doi:10.1186/1751-0147-54-S1-S17

78. Brinkel J, Khan MH, Kraemer A. A systematic review of arsenic exposure and its social and mental health effects with special reference to Bangladesh. *Int J Environ Res Public Health*. 2009;6(5):1609–1619. doi:10.3390/ijerph6051609

79. Kern JK, Geier DA, Bjørklund G, et al. Evidence supporting a link between dental amalgams and chronic illness, fatigue, depression, anxiety, and suicide. Neuro Endocrinol Lett. 2014;35(7):537-52.

80. Troiano G, Mercurio I, Melai P, et al. Suicide behaviour and arsenic levels in drinking water: a possible association?: A review of the literature about the effects of arsenic contamination in drinking water on suicides. *Egypt J Forensic Sci*. 2017;7(1):2. doi:10.1186/s41935-017-0005-y

81. Taki Y, Kinomura S, Sato K, et al. Both global gray matter volume and regional gray matter volume negatively correlate with lifetime alcohol intake in non-alcohol-dependent Japanese men: a volumetric analysis and a voxel-based morphometry. Alcohol Clin Exp Res. 2006;30(6):1045-50. doi:10.1111/j.1530-0277.2006.00118.x

82. Franklin TR, Wetherill RR, Jagannathan K, et al. The effects of chronic cigarette smoking on gray matter volume: influence of sex. *PLoS One*. 2014;9(8):e104102. Published 2014 Aug 4. doi:10.1371/journal.pone.0104102

83. Filbey FM, Aslan S, Calhoun VD, et al. Long-term effects of marijuana use on the brain. PNAS. 2014;111(47):16913-8. doi:10.1073/pnas.1415297111.

84. Orr C, Spechler P, Cao Z, et al. Grey Matter Volume Differences Associated with Extremely Low Levels of Cannabis Use in Adolescence. J Neurosci. 2019;39(10):1817-1827. doi: 10.1523/JNEUROSCI.3375-17.2018.

85. Browning KN, Verheijden S, Boeckxstaens GE. The Vagus Nerve in Appetite Regulation, Mood, and Intestinal Inflammation. *Gastroenterology*. 2016;152(4):730–744. doi:10.1053/j.gastro.2016.10.046

86. David LA, Maurice CF, Carmody RN, et al. Diet rapidly and reproducibly alters the human gut microbiome. *Nature*. 2013;505(7484):559–563. doi:10.1038/nature12820

87. Kahleova H, Belinova L, Malinska H, et al. Eating two larger meals a day (breakfast and lunch) is more effective than six smaller meals in a reduced-energy regimen for patients with type 2 diabetes: a randomised crossover study [published correction appears in Diabetologia. 2015 Jan;58(1):205]. *Diabetologia*. 2014;57(8):1552–1560. doi:10.1007/s00125-014-3253-5

88. Li L, Wang Z, Zuo Z. Chronic intermittent fasting improves cognitive functions and brain structures in mice. *PLoS One*. 2013;8(6):e66069. Published 2013 Jun 3. doi:10.1371/journal.pone.0066069

89. Mullington JM, Simpson NS, Meier-Ewert HK, et al. Sleep loss and inflammation. *Best Pract Res Clin Endocrinol Metab*. 2010;24(5):775–784. doi:10.1016/j.beem.2010.08.014

90. Tabak BA, McCullough ME. Perceived transgressor agreeableness decreases cortisol response and increases forgiveness following recent interpersonal transgressions. Biol Psychol. 2011;87(3):386-92. doi: 10.1016/j.biopsycho.2011.05.001.

91. Fillon M. Holding a Grudge Can Be Bad for Your Health. WebMD. https://www.webmd.com/depression/news/20000225/holding-a-grudge-can-be-bad-for-your-health#2. Published February 25, 2000. Accessed April 23, 2019.

92. McCullough ME, Pedersen EJ, Tabak BA, et al. Conciliatory gestures promote forgiveness and reduce anger in humans. *Proc Natl Acad Sci U S A*. 2014;111(30):11211–11216. doi:10.1073/pnas.1405072111

93. Lupis SB, Lerman M, Wolf JM. Anger responses to psychosocial stress predict heart rate and cortisol stress responses in men but not women. *Psychoneuroendocrinology*. 2014;49:84–95. doi:10.1016/j.psyneuen.2014.07.004

94. Norman K. Forgiveness: How it Manifests in our Health, Well-being, and Longevity. 2017

95. Toussaint L, Shields GS, Dorn G, Slavich GM. Effects of lifetime stress exposure on mental and physical health in young adulthood: How stress degrades and forgiveness protects health. *J Health Psychol*. 2014;21(6):1004–1014. doi:10.1177/1359105314544132

96. Seminowicz DA, Shpaner M, Keaser ML, et al. Cognitive-behavioral therapy increases prefrontal cortex gray matter in patients with chronic pain. *J Pain.* 2013;14(12):1573–1584. doi:10.1016/j.jpain.2013.07.020

97. McCrae CS, Mundt JM, Curtis AF, et al. Gray Matter Changes Following Cognitive Behavioral Therapy for Patients With Comorbid Fibromyalgia and Insomnia: A Pilot Study. *J Clin Sleep Med.* 2018;14(9):1595–1603. doi:10.5664/jcsm.7344

98. Hage MP, Azar ST. The Link between Thyroid Function and Depression. *J Thyroid Res.* 2011;2012:590648. doi:10.1155/2012/590648

99. Chakrabarti S. Thyroid functions and bipolar affective disorder. *J Thyroid Res.* 2011;2011:306367. doi:10.4061/2011/306367

100. Kikuchi M, Komuro R, Oka H, et al. Relationship between anxiety and thyroid function in patients with panic disorder. Prog Neuropsychopharmacol Biol Psychiatry. 2005;29(1):77-81. doi:10.1016/j.pnpbp.2004.10.008

101. Wu H, Hong T, Gao H, et al. Effects of thyroid autoimmunity on pregnancy outcomes in euthyroid women receiving in vitro fertilization: a meta-analysis. Zhonghua Yi Xue Za Zhi. 2015;95(46):3770-4.

102. Unuane D, Velkeniers B, Bravenboer B, et al. Impact of thyroid autoimmunity in euthyroid women on live birth rate after IUI. Hum Reprod. 2017;32(4):915-922. doi: 10.1093/humrep/dex033.

103. He H, Jing S, Gong F, et al. Effect of thyroid autoimmunity per se on assisted reproduction treatment outcomes: A meta-analysis. Taiwan J Obstet Gynecol. 2016;55(2):159-65. doi: 10.1016/j.tjog.2015.09.003.

104. Bliddal S, Nielsen CH, Feldt-Rasmussen U. Recent advances in understanding autoimmune thyroid disease: the tallest tree in the forest of polyautoimmunity. *F1000Res.* 2017;6:1776. Published 2017 Sep 28. doi:10.12688/f1000research.11535.1

105. Wang C. The Relationship between Type 2 Diabetes Mellitus and Related Thyroid Diseases. *J Diabetes Res.* 2013;2013:390534. doi:10.1155/2013/390534

106. Ichiki T. Thyroid hormone and atherosclerosis. Vascul Pharmacol. 2010;52(3-4):151-6. doi: 10.1016/j.vph.2009.09.004.

107. Sanyal D, Raychaudhuri M. Hypothyroidism and obesity: An intriguing link. *Indian J Endocrinol Metab.* 2016;20(4):554–557. doi:10.4103/2230-8210.183454

108. Scott LV, Clarke G, Dinan TG. The brain-gut axis: a target for treating stress-related disorders. Mod Trends Pharmacopsychiatry. 2013;28:90-9. doi: 10.1159/000343971.

109. Messaoudi M, Violle N, Bisson JF, et al. Beneficial psychological effects of a probiotic formulation (Lactobacillus helveticus R0052 and Bifidobacterium longum R0175) in healthy human volunteers. Gut Microbes. 2011;2(4):256-61. doi: 10.4161/gmic.2.4.16108.

110. Farzi A, Fröhlich EE, Holzer P. Gut Microbiota and the Neuroendocrine System. *Neurotherapeutics*. 2018;15(1):5–22. doi:10.1007/s13311-017-0600-5

111. Foster JA, McVey Neufeld KA. Gut-brain axis: how the microbiome influences anxiety and depression. Trends Neurosci. 2013;36(5):305-12. doi: 10.1016/j.tins.2013.01.005.

112. Young-Wolff KC, Alabaster AI, McCaw B, et al. Adverse Childhood Experiences and Mental and Behavioral Health Conditions During Pregnancy: The Role of Resilience. J Womens Health (Larchmt). 2019;28(4):452-61. doi: 10.1089/jwh.2018.7108.

113. Seidelmann SB, Claggett B, Cheng S, Henglin M, Shah A, Steffen LM, Folsom AR, Rimm EB, Willett WC, Solomon SD. Dietary carbohydrate intake and mortality: a prospective cohort study and meta-analysis. *Lancet Public Health*. 2018;3(9):e419–e428.

114. Melina V, Craig W, Levin S. Position of the academy of nutrition and dietetics: Vegetarian diets. *J Acad Nutr Diet*. 2016;116(12):1970-1980.

115. Condé Nast. Foods. SELF Nutrition Data: Know What You Eat. https://nutritiondata.self.com/ Accessed October 8, 2019.

116. Noah ND, Bender AE, Reaidi GB, Gilbert RJ. Food poisoning from raw red kidney beans. *Br Med J*. 1980;281(6234):236-7.

117. Rodhouse JC, Haugh CA, Roberts D, Gilbert RJ. Red kidney bean poisoning in the UK: an analysis of 50 suspected incidents between 1976 and 1989. *Epidemiol Infect*. 1990;105(3):485-91.

118. Pusztai A, Grant G. Assessment of lectin inactivation by heat and digestion. *Methods in Molecular Medicine. Methods Mol Med*. 1998;9:505-14.

119. Pal RS, Bhartiya A, Yadav P, Kant L, Mishra KK, Aditya JP, Pattanayak A. Effect of dehulling, germination and cooking on nutrients, anti-nutrients,

fatty acid composition and antioxidant properties in lentil (Lens culinaris). *J Food Sci Technol.* 2017;54(4):909-20.

120. Navert B, Sandstrom B, Cederblad A. Reduction of the Phytate Content of Bran by Leavening in Bread and Its Effect on Zinc-Absorption in Man. *Br J Nutr.* 1985;53(1):47-53.

121. Lajolo F, Genovese M. Nutritional Significance of Lectins and Enzyme Inhibitors from Legumes. *J Agric Food Chem.* 2002;50(22):6592-8.

122. Gibson RS, Heath AL, Szymlek-Gay EA. Is iron and zinc nutrition a concern for vegetarian infants and young children in industrialized countries? *Am J Clin Nutr.* 2014 Jul;100 Suppl 1:459S-68S.

123. Rizzo NS, Jaceldo-Siegl K, Sabate J, Fraser GE. Nutrient profiles of vegetarian and non-vegetarian dietary patterns. *J Acad Nutr Diet.* 2013;113(12):1610-9.

124. Burckhardt P. The role of low acid load in vegetarian diet on bone health: A narrative review. *Swiss Med Wkly.* 2016;146:w14277.

125. Kim YJ, Chung HY. Antioxidative and anti-inflammatory actions of docosahexaenoic acid and eicosapentaenoic acid in renal epithelial cells and macrophages. *J Med Food.* 2007;10(2):225-31.

126. Burdge GC, Jones AE, Wootton SA. Eicosapentaenoic and docosapentaenoic acids are the principal products of α-linolenic acid metabolism in young men. *Br J Nutr.* 2002;88(4):355-364.

127. Burdge GC, Wootton SA. Conversion of α-linolenic acid to eicosapentaenoic, docosapentaenoic and docosahexaenoic acids in young women. *Br J Nutr.* 2002;88(4):411-420.

128. Litalien C, Beaulieu P. Chapter 117 - Molecular Mechanisms of Drug Actions: From Receptors to Effectors, In *Pediatric Critical Care* (Fourth Edition), edited by Bradley P. Fuhrman and Jerry J. Zimmerman, Mosby, Saint Louis, 2011, Pages 1553-1568, ISBN 9780323073073, 10.1016/B978-0-323-07307-3.10117-X.

129. Beezhold BL, Johnston CS. Restriction of meat, fish, and poultry in omnivores improves mood: a pilot randomized controlled trial." *Nutr J.* 2012;11:9.

130. Adam O, Tesche A, et al. Impact of linoleic acid intake on arachidonic acid formation and eicosanoid biosynthesis in humans. *Prostaglandins Leukot Essent Fatty Acids.* 2008;79(3-5):177-81.

131. Simopoulos AP. The importance of the ratio of omega-6/omega-3 essential fatty acids. *Biomed Pharmacother.* 2002;56(8):365-79.

132. Saunders AV, Davis BC, Garg ML. Omega-3 polyunsaturated fatty acids and vegetarian diets. *Med J Aust.* 2013;199(S4):S22-6.

133. Rodriguez-Leyva D, Dupasquier CM, McCullough R, Pierce GN. The cardiovascular effects of flaxseed and its omega-3 fatty acid, alpha-linolenic acid. Can J Cardiol. 2010;26(9):489-96.

134. Food and Nutrition Board, Institute of Medicine. Dietary Fats: Total Fat and Fatty Acids. Dietary Reference Intakes for Energy, Carbohydrate, Fiber, Fat, Fatty Acids, Cholesterol, Protein, and Amino Acids. Washington, D.C.: National Academies Press; 2002:422-541.

135. Zeilmaker MJ, Hoekstra J, van Eijkeren JC, de Jong N, Hart A, Kennedy M, Owen H, Gunnlaugsdottir H. Fish consumption during child bearing age: A quantitative risk–benefit analysis on neurodevelopment. *Food Chem Toxicol.* 2013;54:30-4.

136. Glynn A, Aune M, Darnerud PO, Cnattingius S, Bjerselius R, Becker W, Lignell S. Determinants of serum concentrations of organochlorine compounds in Swedish pregnant women: A cross-sectional study. *Environ Health.* 2007;6:2.

137. Ginde AA, Liu MC, Camargo CA Jr.. Demographic Differences and Trends of Vitamin D Insufficiency in the US Population, 1988-2004." Arch Intern Med. 2009;169(6):626-32.

138. Johnson LE. "Vitamin B 12 - Disorders of Nutrition - Merck Manuals Consumer Version." Merck Manuals Professional Edition, Merck Manual, merckmanuals.com/home/disorders-of-nutrition/vitamins/vitamin-b-12.

ABOUT THE AUTHOR

DR. JANELLE LOUIS IS a Vermont-licensed naturopathic doctor who specializes in helping people who have experienced traumatic events during childhood overcome the health concerns they are at increased risk for as a result, including mental health conditions, reproductive concerns, autoimmune diseases, and metabolic syndrome. Dr. Louis is committed to ensuring that her clients live their healthiest lives now in spite of their difficult pasts.

She is the author of Set On Edge and Optimize Your Body, Heal Your Mind and developer of the B.A.L.A.N.C.E. Framework™ and the P7 Protocol™ for integrated mental wellness. Dr. Louis is currently engaged in private practice at Focus Integrative Healthcare in Atlanta, Georgia where she helps people regain optimal overall wellbeing by addressing a variety of physical and mental health concerns. Dr. Louis enjoys providing exceptional, person-focused care to individuals from all walks of life. Her clients appreciate her ability to apply her knowledge of both pharmaceutical medication and natural therapeutics to their unique situations in order to help them reach their health goals. She loves helping people to optimize their health naturally and to live radiantly!

When she is not in her private practice, Dr. Louis enjoys spending time with her husband and sons, writing, teaching, traveling, and camping.

- ATTENTION CHILDHOOD TRAUMA SURVIVORS -

FAMILY CURSES ARE REAL: FIND OUT HOW YOUR PARENTS' EXPERIENCES AND TRAUMA ARE AFFECTING YOU EVEN NOW

Download my FREE bonus chapter to learn the good news about getting rid of your genetic baggage today!

You can't shake that nagging feeling. Nobody had to tell you for you to know. Something's wrong. There just has to be something wrong with some of the genes (I'm talking DNA) passed down in your family. You may know that your childhood trauma is making it a struggle to achieve "normal" mental and physical health. What you may not know is that your parents' past trauma and experiences, even before you were born, can affect you (physically and mentally) as an adult. It's unbelievably profound! It can even reach back to Grandma and Grandpa.

Finding out HOW will be an empowering experience. It's in the HOW that you'll see the way to break the curse. Read this special bonus chapter, "Overcoming My Family Curse: The What and How," today. This information didn't make it into the book before its release, but it's so vital I'm making it available to download (on a special website) today for FREE. You'll discover how it happens and how you can take advantage of that knowledge to form a plan to stop the curse in its tracks. Enough is enough. Download my FREE bonus chapter today to stop the curse by going to —

www.AceDefyers.com/bonus-chapter

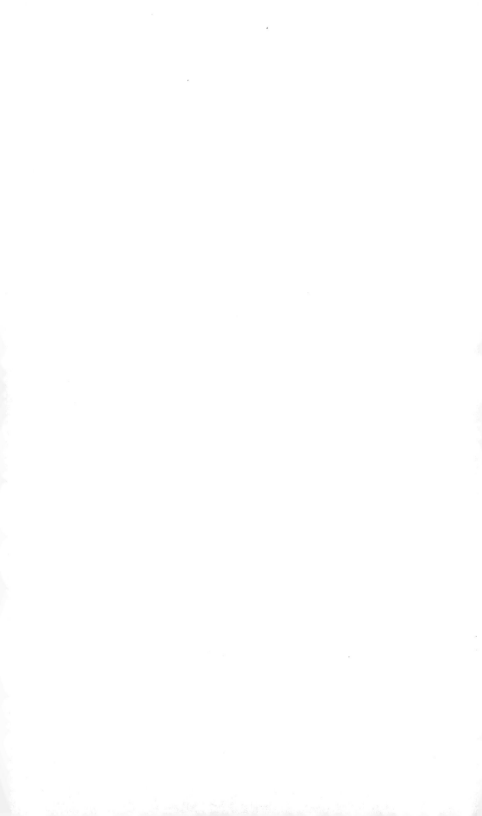

Printed in Poland
by Amazon Fulfillment
Poland Sp. z o.o., Wrocław

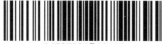